Mediterranean Diet Cookbook For Beginners

Delicious and Healthy Recipes to Weight Loss

Ben Cooper

Table of contents

Italian Meatball Soup

Preparation Time: 10 minutes
Cooking Time: 45 minutes
Servings: 6

Ingredients:

1/4 - 1/2 cup freshly grated parmesan cheese (optional)
1 free-range egg
1 cup breadcrumbs, optional
2 tbsp. fresh parsley, minced
1 tsp. dried oregano
1/2 tsp. sea salt
½ tsp. black pepper
3 tbsp. olive oil
2 quarts chicken broth or beef broth
3 tbsp. tomato paste
1 onion, diced
2 bay leaves
4-5 sprigs fresh thyme
½ tsp. whole black peppercorns
Fresh parmesan cheese, grated 1-2 tbsp.
Fresh basil leaves, torn
1-2 tbsp. fresh parsley, chopped
Salt and pepper, to taste

Directions:

1.Place all the meatball ingredients except the oil into a medium bowl.

2.Using your hands, mix well and form into meatballs.

3.Place the oil into a stock pot, place over a medium heat and add the meatballs, browning on all sides.

4.Remove the meatballs from the pan.

5.Add more oil to the pan if needed and then add the onion. Cook for five minutes until soft.

6.Add the remaining soup ingredients, stir well then cook for 10 minutes.

7.Return the meatballs to the pan and simmer for a few minutes to warm through.

8.Serve and enjoy.

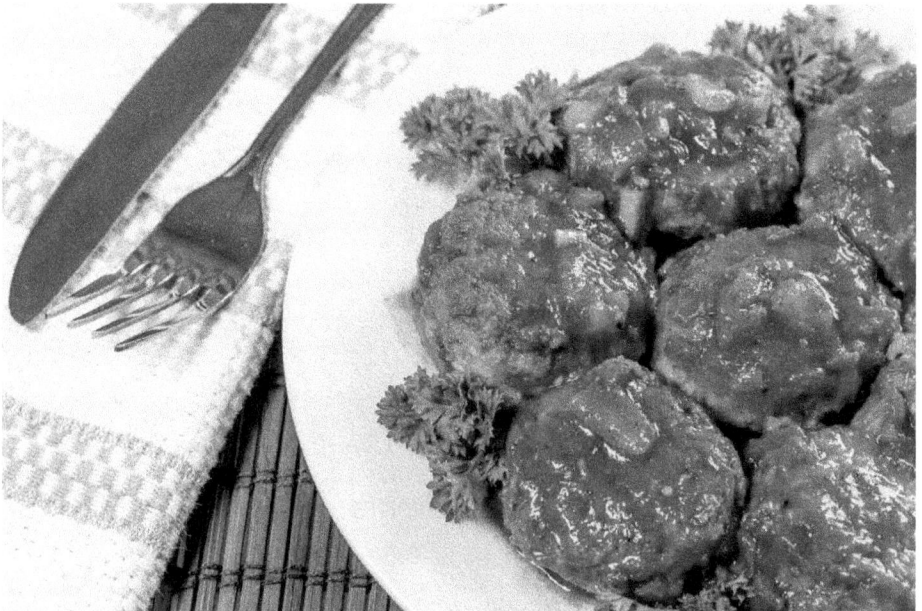

Tuscan White Bean Soup with Sausage and Kale

Preparation Time: 10 minutes

Cooking Time: 40 minutes

Servings: 6

Ingredients:

¼ cup extra virgin olive oil 1 lb. hot sausage,
1 onion, chopped
1 carrot, chopped
1 stalk celery, chopped
2 cloves garlic, chopped
½ lb. kale, stems removed and chopped
4 cups chicken broth
1 x 28 oz. can cannelloni beans, rinsed and drained
1 tsp. rosemary, dried
1 bay leaf
Pepper Salt, to taste
½ cup shredded parmesan

Directions:

1.Find a stock pot, pop over a medium heat and add the oil.

2.Cook the sausage until browned on all sides.

3.Throw in the onion, carrot, celery and garlic then cook for a further five minutes.

4.Add the kale and stir through.

5.Next add the broth, beans, rosemary and bay leaf.

6.Stir well, bring to the boil then cover with the lid.

7.Turn down the heat then simmer for 30 minutes.

8.Serve and enjoy.

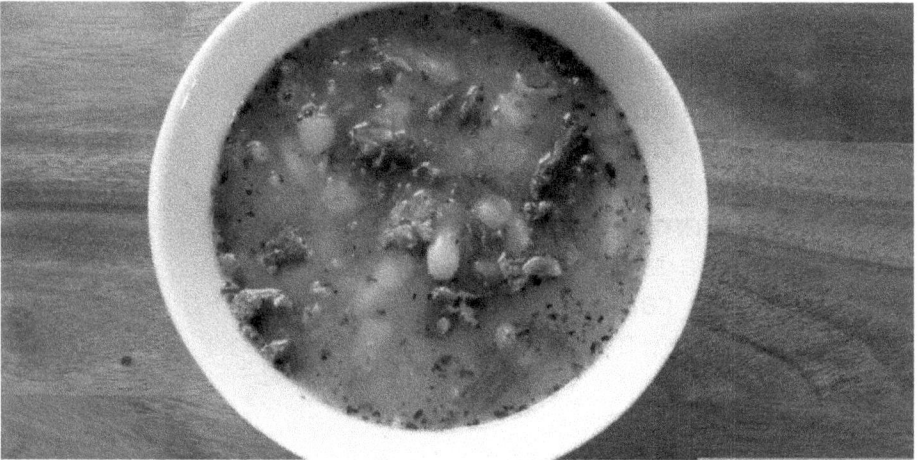

Vegetable Soup

Preparation Time: 10 minutes
Cooking Time: 45 minutes
Servings: 4

Ingredients:

Extra virgin olive oil, to taste
8 oz. sliced baby Bella mushrooms
2 medium-size zucchinis, sliced
1 bunch flat leaf parsley, chopped
1 red onion, chopped
2 garlic cloves, chopped
2 celery ribs, chopped
2 carrots, peeled, chopped
2 golden potatoes, peeled, diced
1 tsp. ground coriander
1/2 tsp. turmeric powder
1/2 tsp. sweet paprika
1/2 tsp. thyme
Salt and pepper
1 x 32 oz. can whole peeled tomatoes 2 bay leaves
6 cups turkey or vegetable broth
1 x 15 oz. can garbanzo beans, rinsed and drained Juice
and zest of 1 lime
1/3 cup toasted pine nuts, optional

Directions:

1.Grab a large stockpot, add a tbsp. of olive oil and pop over a medium heat.

2.Add the mushrooms and cook for five minutes, stirring often.

3.Remove from the pan and pop to one side.

4.Add the sliced zucchini and cook for another five minutes. Remove from the pan.

5.Add more oil and add the parsley, onions, garlic, celery, carrots and potatoes. Stir through the spices, salt and pepper.

6.Cook for five minutes until the veggies are softening.

7.Add the tomatoes, bay leaves and broth then bring to a boil.

8.Cover and cook on medium low for 15 minutes.

9.Remove the lid and add the garbanzo beans, mushrooms and zucchini.

10.Heat then serve and enjoy.

Sweet Yogurt Bulgur Bowl

Preparation Time: 10 minutes

Cooking Time: 0 minutes

Servings: 4

Ingredients:
1 cup grapes, halved
½ cup bulgur, cooked
¼ cup celery stalk, chopped
2 oz walnuts, chopped
¼ cup plain yogurt
½ tsp. ground cinnamon

Directions:

1.Mix grapes with bulgur, celery stalk, and walnut

2.Then add plain yogurt and ground cinnamon.

3.Stir the mixture with the help of the spoon and transfer in the serving bowls.

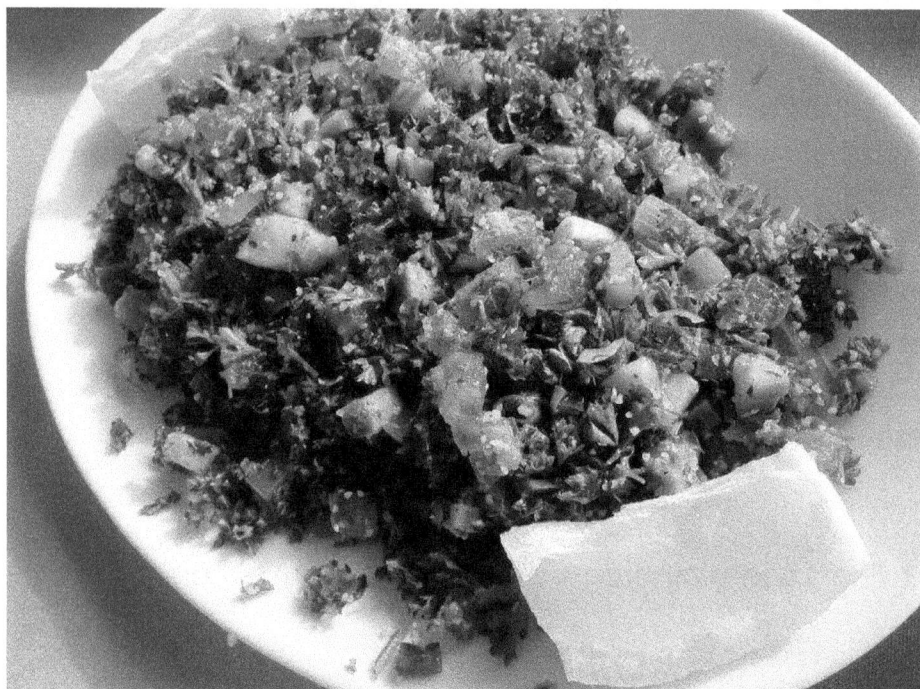

Spring Farro Plate

Preparation Time: 15 minutes

Cooking Time: 0 minutes

Servings: 6

Ingredients:

1 cup farro, cooked
2 cups baby spinach
2 grapefruits, roughly chopped
2 tbsp. balsamic vinegar
¼ tsp. white pepper
1 tbsp. olive oil

Directions:

1.Mix baby spinach and farro in the big bowl.

2.Then add grapefruit and shake the ingredients well.

3.Transfer the mixture in the serving plates and sprinkle with white pepper, olive oil, and balsamic vinegar.

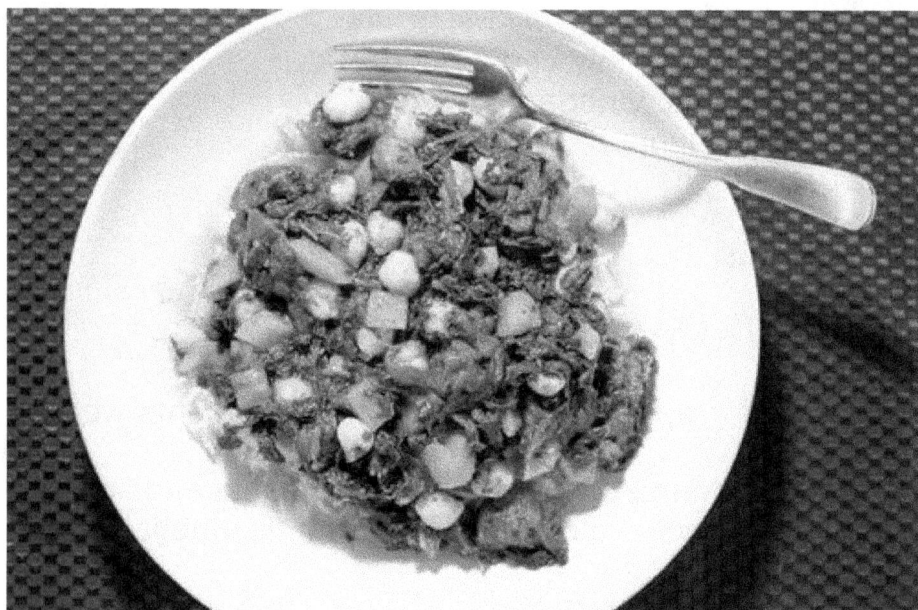

Sorghum Taboule

Preparation Time: 10 minutes
Cooking Time: 0 minutes
Servings: 2

Ingredients:

2 oz sorghum, cooked
3 oz pumpkin, diced, boiled
½ white onion, diced 1 date, pitted, chopped
1 tbsp. avocado oil
½ tsp. liquid honey
2 oz Feta, crumbled

Directions:

1.Put sorghum, pumpkin, onion, and date in the big bowl.

2.Then sprinkle the ingredients with avocado oil and liquid honey. Stir well.

3.Transfer the cooked taboule in the serving plates and top with crumbled feta.

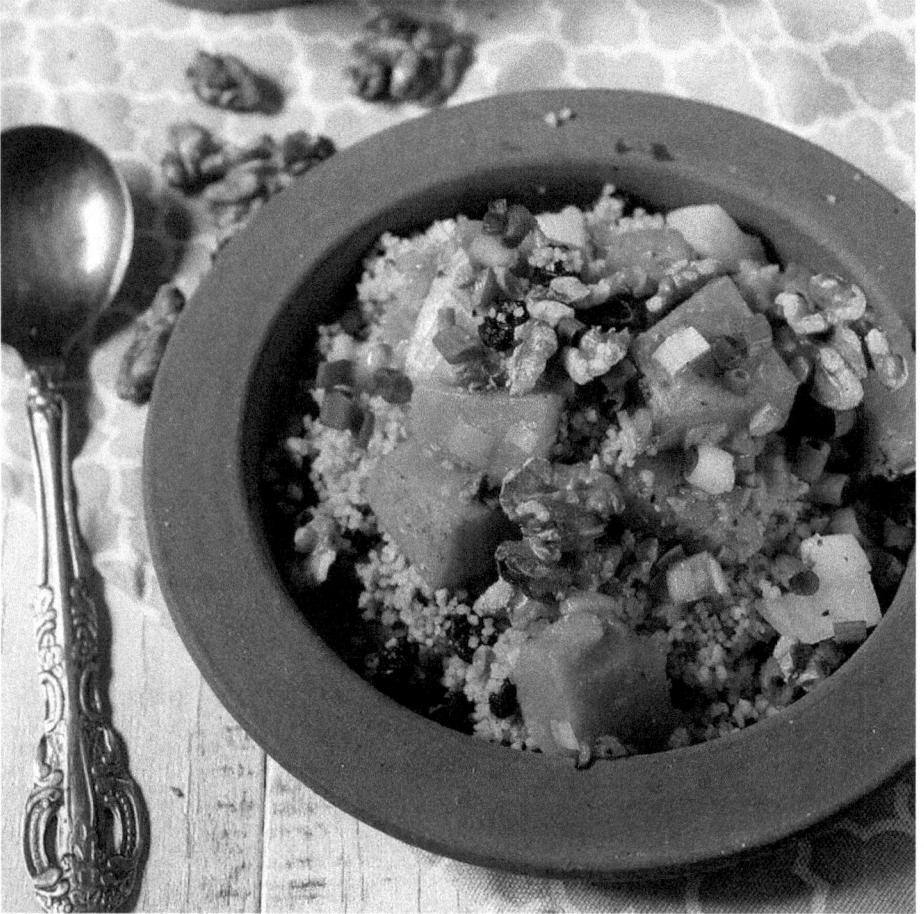

Roasted Vegetable soup

Preparation Time: 10 minutes

Cooking Time: 45 minutes

Servings: 6

Ingredients:

2 cups Vegetable stock; 2 cups
2 sliced red bell pepper
4 tomatoes; diced
2 cups of water
A sprig of rosemary
Olive oil; 3 tablespoons
1 sliced carrot
2 red onions; cut in halves
4 cloves
Pepper and salt to taste
A small butternut; crushed, peeled and diced

Directions:

1.Get a baking tray and add your carrot, cloves, tomatoes, red onions, parsnip, bell pepper, rosemary and crushed butternut.

2.Add pepper and salt to taste then drizzle with oil

3.Now, preheat your oven to 350F, then cook for 25-30 minutes till it turns golden brown.

4.Move your vegetable into a soup pot and add in the stock and some water then cook for another 10 minutes.

5.After 10 minutes, remove the rosemary then grind with an immersion blender.

6.Enjoy your soup when warm.

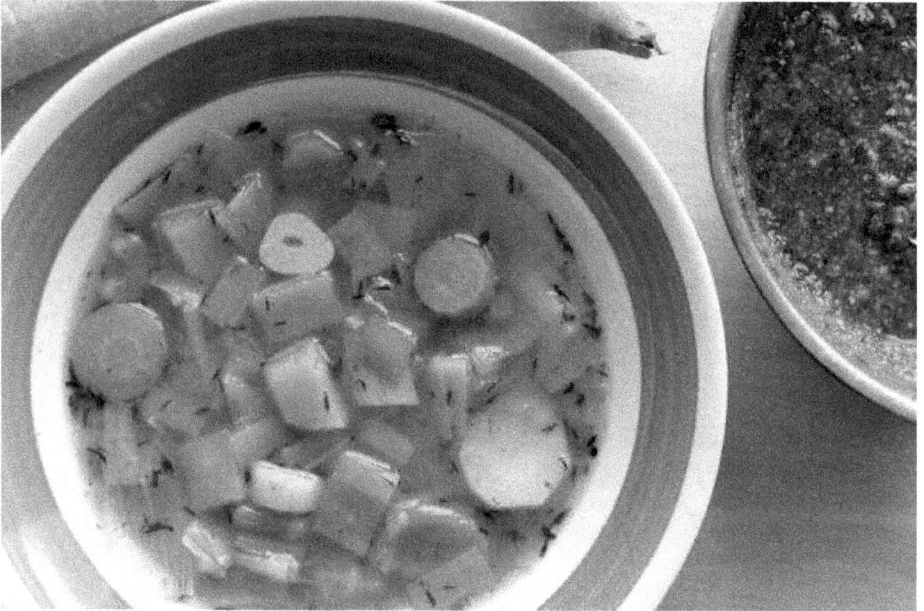

Mediterranean Chicken Soup

Preparation Time: 10 minutes

Cooking Time: 30 minutes

Servings: 4

Ingredients:

2 sliced cloves
2 peeled and sliced tomatoes
A bay leaf
1 juiced lemon
1 sweet onion; diced
1 cubed zucchini
Water; 4 cups
½ teaspoon of capers; sliced
½ teaspoon of oregano; dried
Dried basil; 1 teaspoon
½ cup of orzo
2 cups Chicken stock
1 pound of chicken drumsticks
1 chopped and cored green bell pepper
1 chopped and cored red bell pepper
Pepper and salt to taste

Directions:

1.Get a soup pot and add your vegetable, stock, herbs, chicken, bay leaf and water together, then add pepper and salt to taste and cook on low heat for 25 minutes.

2.Now add your lemon juice and cook again for 5 minutes.

3.Serve and enjoy your warm soup.

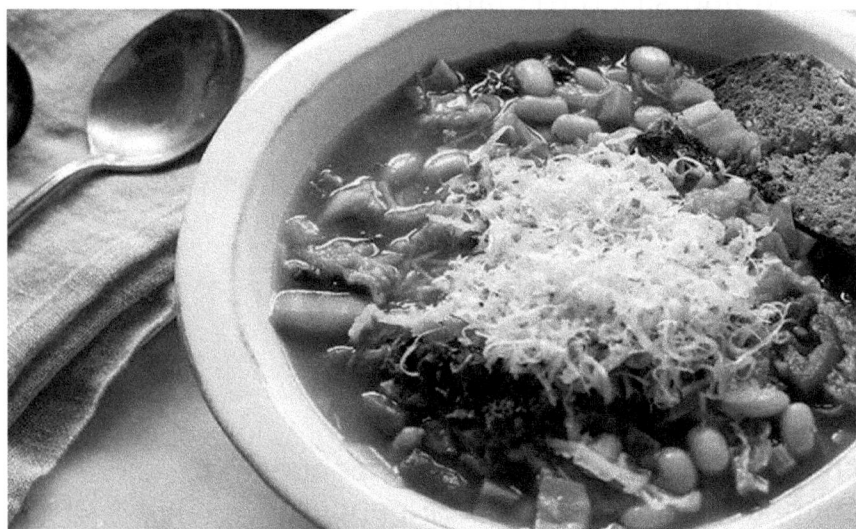

Mediterranean Bean and Sausage soup

Preparation Time: 10 minutes

Cooking Time: 30 minutes

Servings: 4

Ingredients:

2 tbsp Olive oil; 2 tablespoons
A can of drained black beans
1 cup Juiced tomato; 1 cup
4 cups of water
1 pound of sliced chicken sausage
2 cups of chicken stalk
1 chopped celery stalk
2 sliced cloves
1 can of drained kidney beans
1 sliced carrot
2 peeled and sliced tomatoes
A rosemary sprig
1 bay leaf
A sweet onion; diced
Pepper and salt to taste

Directions:

1.Get a soup pot and heat your olive oil, then pour in your sausage and cook for 5 minutes.

2.Now, add all other Ingredients

3.Add pepper and salt to taste and cook for 25 minutes.

4.Serve and enjoy when cooled

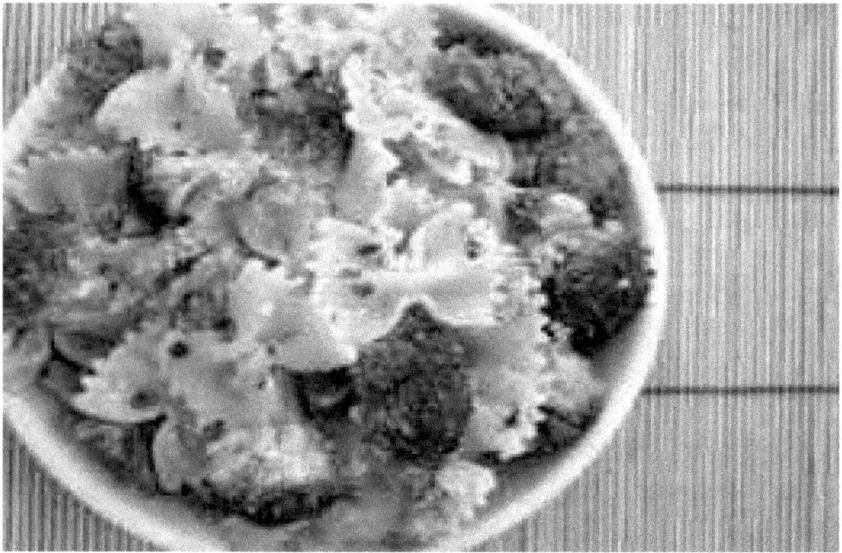

Spicy Avocado soup

Preparation Time: 10 minutes

Cooking Time: 25 minutes

Servings:4

Ingredients:

2 tablespoons of olive oil
1 cored and sliced red pepper
2 peeled and sliced avocado
4 cups Water; 4 cups
A sprig of thyme
2 cups Baby spinach; 2 cups
A sprig of oregano
2 sliced cloves
1 sliced celery stalk
2 cups of vegetable stock
1 sliced shallot
¼ cup of sliced cilantro
1 chopped jelapeno
Pepper and salt to taste

Directions:

1.Get a soup pot and heat your olive oil, then pour in your sliced celery, clove, oregano, shallot, red pepper and thyme.

2.Now, pour in your chopped jelapeno, stock and water then add pepper and salt to taste and cook on low heat for 10 minutes.

3.Add your spinach and cook for 10 minutes again.

4.Now, pour the soup into serving bowls and add your avocado and cilantro slice on top.

5.Serve and enjoy.

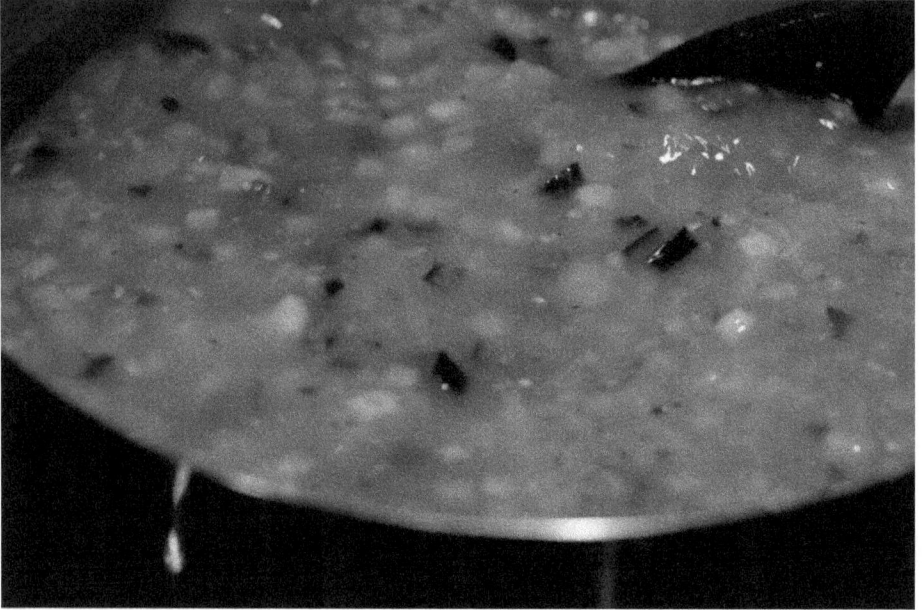

Smoked Ham and Split Pea soup

Preparation Time: 10 minutes

Cooking Time: 35 minutes

Servings:4

Ingredients:

Water; 6 cups
½ cup of split pea
1 sliced jalapeno pepper
4 Oz of diced smoked ham
2 carrots; chopped
2 tomatoes; peeled and sliced
1 diced sweet onion
1 sliced parsnip
2 cups of vegetable stock
1 juiced lemon
Olive oil; 2 tablespoons
2 carrots; sliced
2 cloves; sliced
2 red bell pepper; cored and sliced
Creme fraiche to serve

Directions:

1.Get a soup pot and heat your olive oil, then pour in your ham and cook for 5 minutes, then pour the rest of your ingredients.

2.Add pepper and salt to taste, then cook for 30 minutes with low heat.

3.Serve your warm soup topped with creme fraiche and enjoy.

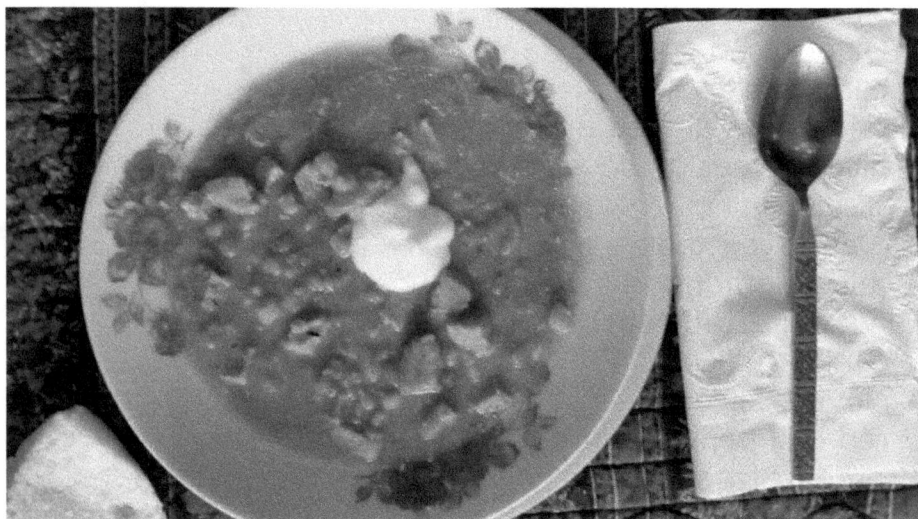

Mediterranean Beef Toss Spaghetti

Total time - 25 min
Servings - 4

Ingredients:

½ pound Lean ground beef
¾ tsp Divided salt
¼ tsp Pepper
1 Medium red onion, sliced
1-inch pieces - 1Medium green pepper, cut into 1-inch pieces
1 can Diced tomatoes, undrained
1 tsp Red wine vinegar
1 tsp Dried basil
1 tsp Dried thyme
2 medium zucchinis, sliced
3 tbsp of olive oil, divided
4 garlic cloves, minced
Hot cooked spaghetti (optional)

Directions:

1.Cook the beef, garlic, 1 4 teaspoon salt and pepper in 1 teaspoon oil in a nonstick pan over medium heat until meat is no longer pink

2.Drain the pan after the meat has cooked.

3.Empty the pan into a bowl and keep warm.

4.Sauté the onion in oil for 2 minutes using the same pan.

5.Pour zucchini and green pepper into the pan, and stir continuously for 4-6 minutes or until vegetables are crispy soft.

6.Add tomatoes, vinegar, basil, thyme and remaining salt (½ teaspoon) and mix properly.

7.Add beef mixture and heat properly.

8.Serve with spaghetti.

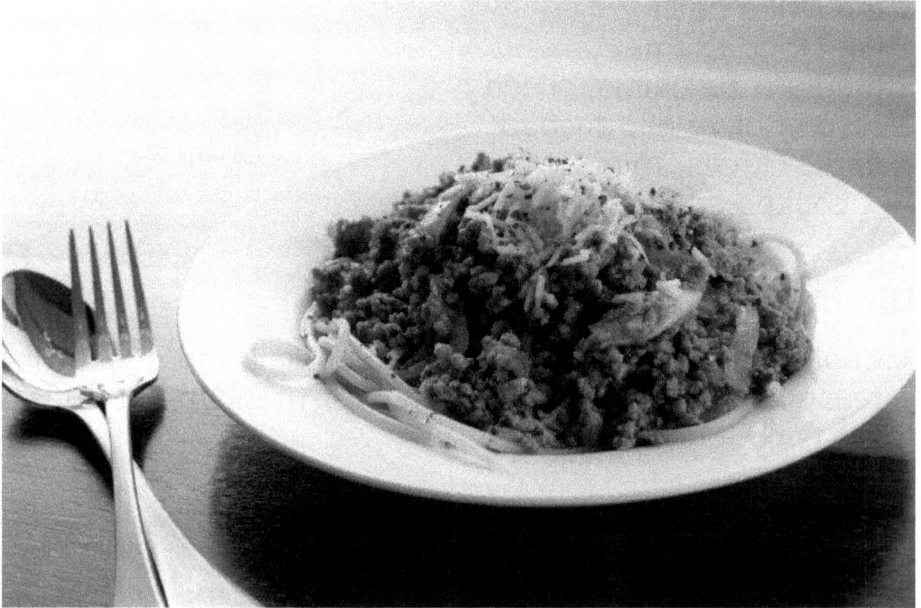

Herb crusted Mediterranean pork tenderloin

Total time – 35 Minutes
Servings - 3

Ingredients:

¾ Pork tenderloin
¾ tbsp Olive oil
½ tsp Dried oregano
1 tsp Lemon pepper
2 tbps Olive tapenade (refrigerated mixed)
¾ ounce Feta cheese (finely crumbled, about 3 tablespoons)

Directions:

1.Put pork on a large plastic wrapper.

2.Apply oil over the tenderloin; sprinkle oregano and lemon pepper all over the surface.

3.Tightly wind the plastic wrapper around the meat; leave in the freezer for 2 hours or overnight.

4.Start a medium heat fire in the grill.

5.Remove meat from plastic wrapper and make a vertical cut through the middle. Do not cut completely through to the opposite side.

6.Open both halves of the meat and apply a generous amount of olive tapénade on one half — Scatter cheese all over the surface.

7.Fold the other half to form the natural shape of tenderloin.

8.Bind tightly with thin cord set 1½ to 2-inches apart.

9.Place the tenderloin over direct heat from the grill for 20 minutes, or the internal temperature reaches 145° F. Remember to switch the sides halfway into the grilling.

10.Move the tenderloin to the cutting board. Cover gently with foil and leave it for 5-10 minutes.

11.Remove the cord and cut into smaller pieces about 1 4-inch-thick

12.Ready to serve

Mediterranean Grilled Pork Roast

Total time - 85 Minutes
Servings – 5

Ingredients:

3/3 pound Pork loin roast, boneless
½ Lemons
4 Garlic (peeled)
¼ cup Rosemary leaves (fresh)
¼ cup Sage leaves (fresh)
¼cup Black pepper (coarsely ground)
7 tbsp Salt

Directions:

1.Gently tap pork roast until it is dry.

2.Put the other Ingredients: in a food processor until you have a beautiful mixture.

3.Apply the processed mixture all over the surface of the pork roast

4.Set grill on medium heat and place the pork to cook over indirect heat.

5.Close the hood and leave it to grill for about 60-80 minutes (20 minutes pound), until internal temperature on the thermometer measures 145° F.

6.Turn off the grill and leave to cool for 10 minutes

7.Cut into smaller slices and serve

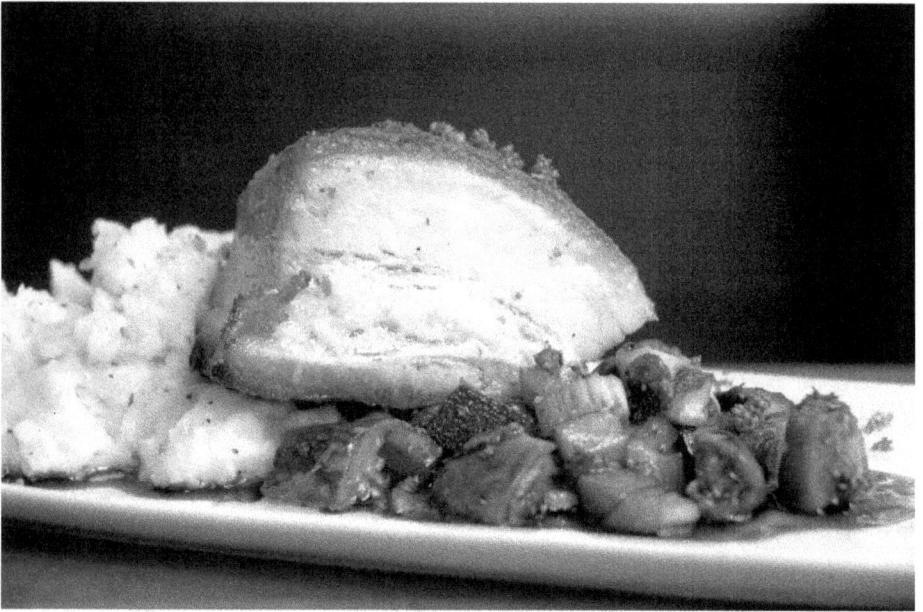

Mediterranean Boneless Pork Kabobs

Total time – 30 Minutes
Servings – 5

Ingredients:

1 ¼ Boneless pork loin (or 4 boneless pork chops)
7 ½ Marinated artichoke hearts
1 ½ Red bell pepper (seeded and cut into 1-inch squares)
11/4 tsp Hot pepper sauce
1 ¼ tsp Oregano
2 ½ tbsp Lemon juice
2 ½ tsp Black pepper

Directions:

1.Dice the pork loin or chops into 1-inch cubes and keep them inside a self-seal cellophane bag.

2.Remove fluids from artichoke hearts while sparing the marinade

3.Put artichoke hearts and bell pepper squares in a separate bowl.

4.Add the remaining Ingredients: and the reserved marinade to the cellophane bag; shake properly and close the bag.

5.Leave it for about 30 minutes while switching the bag's sides regularly (or refrigerate overnight).

6.Set grill to medium heat using coals and covered grill; grill pork on a spit for 15 minutes and artichoke hearts

and pepper squares until well cooked and evenly
browned.

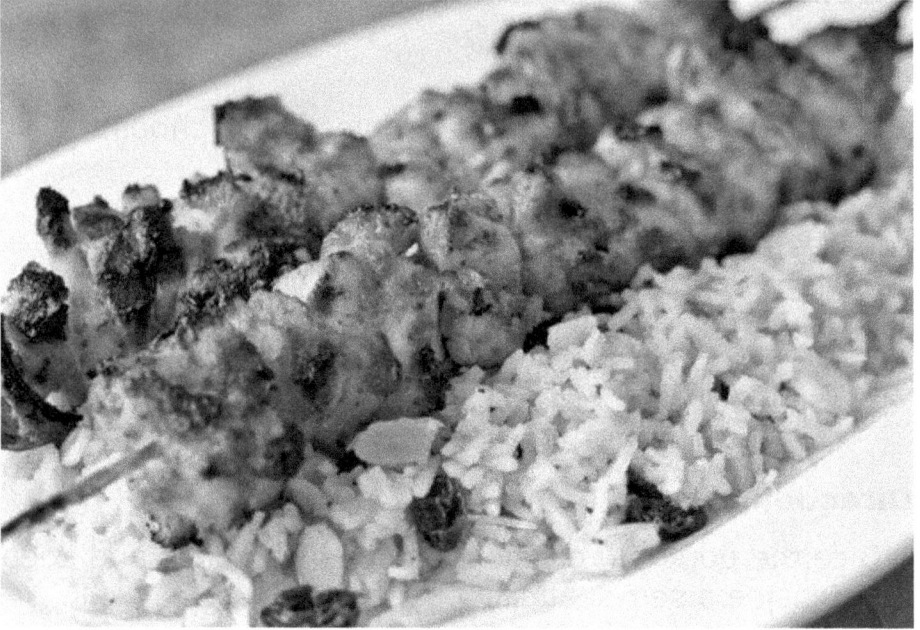

Marinated Mediterranean Grilled Steak

Preparation time - 50 Minutes
Servings – 6

Ingredients:

1 ½ pounds Steak
½ cup Wish-bone (Italian or Robusto-Italian dressing) -
½ cup
2 cloves Finely chopped garlic
2 tsp Sprigs fresh rosemary, torn into pieces teaspoons

Directions:

1.Mix Wish-Bone Italian Dressing, garlic and rosemary to make your marinade.

2.Soak steak in the shallow nonaluminum baking dish or plastic bag and mix properly

3.Close the bowl or bag and leave to marinate for about 30 minutes in the freezer.

4.Remove steak from marinade and throw out the marinade. Keep the unused marinade in the freezer.

5.Grill steak normally, switching sides and brushing regularly with the marinade you kept in the freezer.

6.Continue until steak is done to your satisfaction.

7.Cut into smaller sizes; ready to serve.

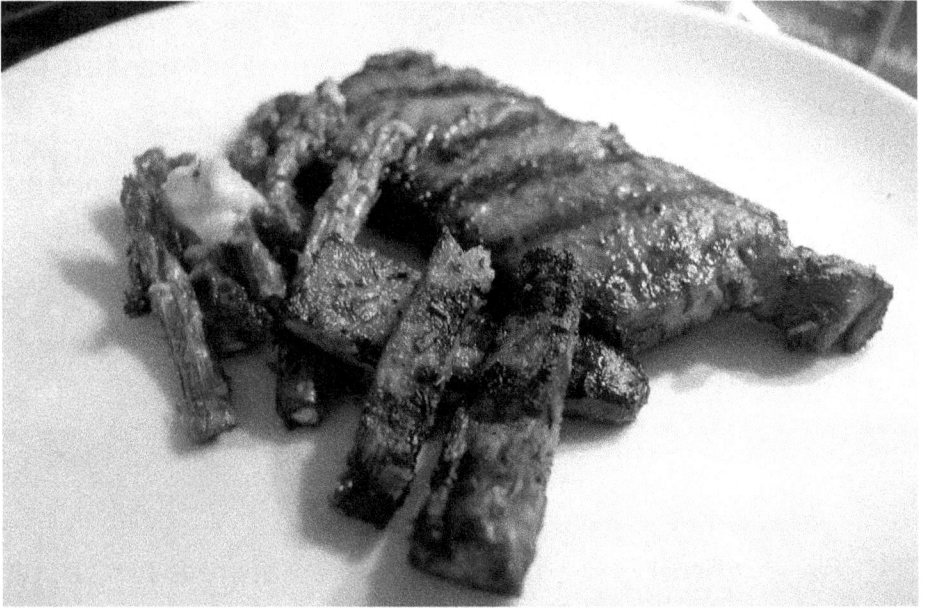

Mediterranean Baked Chicken Skillet

Total time - 40Minutes
Servings – 5

Ingredients:

¼ cup Black olives (sliced)
Black pepper
2 pounds Boneless skinless chicken breasts (organic)
½ tsp Coriander
Crushed red pepper (to taste)
1 ½ cups Diced tomatoes (with the juice)
2 tbsp Feta cheese
2 cloves Garlic (sliced)
2 tbsp Ghee (or olive oil)
1 tsp Onion powder
½ tsp Paprika
Salt
1 cup Yellow onion (chopped)

Directions:

1.First warm oven up to 400ºF.

2.While you wait, mix chicken and onion powder, coriander, paprika, crushed red pepper, salt, and pepper in a bowl.

3.Pour oil into a moderately sized pan and set over medium to high heat.

4.Sauté the chicken until it turns brown and removes from the pan into a separate bowl (not thoroughly cooked, just brown).

5.Cook onions for about 3-5 minutes, garlic for 30 seconds, add diced tomatoes and stir properly.

6.Return the chicken into the pan.

7.Put the pan in the warm oven and leave it to bake for about 20 minutes or until the thermometer reads an internal temperature of 165ºF.

8.Enjoy with black olives and feta cheese topping.

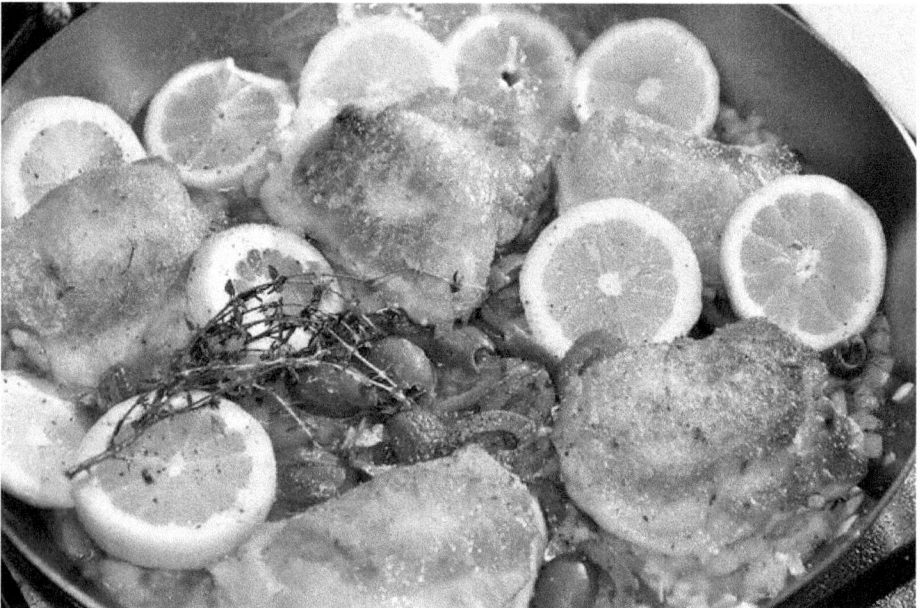

Winter Minestrone

Preparation time: 35 minutes
Cooking time: 60 minutes
Servings: 6

Ingredients:

2 cups chopped cabbage
1 cup chopped cauliflower florets chopped butternut
squash
½ cup chopped onion
½ cup chopped carrot
½ cup diced celery
8 cups water
½ black beans
5 oz small macaroni
¼ grated Parmesan cheese
¼ olive oil Salt to taste
Black pepper to taste

Directions:

1.Mix all the vegetables chopped in a Dutch oven or
large pot. Stir fry for two minutes.

2.Cover it up with water and set it above medium-high
heat.

3.Add in the macaroni, grated cheese, olive oil, and beans.
Bring it to a boil.

4.Lessen the heat to cook and simmer for one hour.

5. Add season as needed with pepper, salt, and extra cheese
if preferred. The soup must be thick.

6.Present in bowls with a garnishing of grated cheese on top of it.

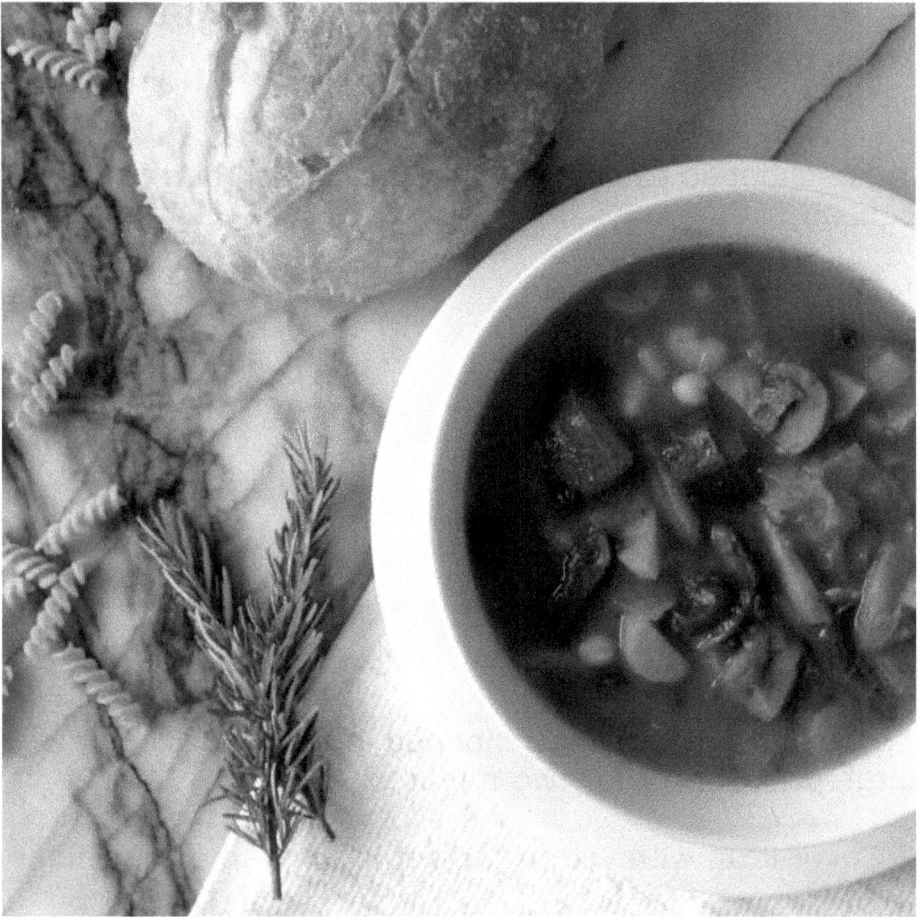

Venezuelan Corn Fritter (Arepas)

Preparation time: 20 minutes
Cooking time: 25 minutes
Servings: 12

Ingredients:
2 corn
2 sliced scallions
1 sliced jalapeño
1/3 cup yellow cornmeal
½ cup flour
1 tsp sugar
¼ tsp salt
½ tsp baking soda
2 tbsp butter
1 egg
½ cup whole milk
2.5 cup canola oil
1 bunch of Papallo leaves
¼ cup sour cream

Directions:

1.Take a large pot; boil enough water to cover the corns.

2.Add corns and cook for five min until they are tender. Cool them, and then into a mixing bowl, slice off the kernels.

3.Add flour, scallions, cornmeal, jalapeños, sugar, baking soda, and salt to the bowl.

4.In a small saucepan, melt the butter, whisk the melted butter, milk, and egg together in another separate bowl. Pour this mixture into the dry ingredients and blend well.

5.Over medium-high heat, add and Heat oil in a large skillet. Add a heaping tbsp of corn batter in oil and spread it to make a pancake of three and a half inches across.

6.Cook it until it is set on one side, then turn over and continue until it turns light brown. Two to three min on each side.

7.Sap on paper towels.

8.Repeat this process until all the batter is gone. Add extra oil, if needed.

9.Dish out with a little crème Fraiche in the core of pancake, if needed, and dust with a cilantro leaf. Enjoy!

Broccoli Cauliflower Carrot Bake

Preparation time: 5 minutes
Cooking time: 50 minutes
Servings: 12

Ingredients:

2 cups broccoli
1cup carrots
2 cups cauliflower
4 tbsp butter
2 tbsp flour
Once pinch of pepper
1 cup of milk
1 cup chopped onions
3 oz softened cream cheese
½ cup shredded sharp cheddar cheese
½ cup soft bread crumbs

Directions:

1.Heat oven at 350 degrees prior.

2.Wash and dice vegetables; steam until they are crisp
but tender, and drain them.

3.Melt two tbsp of butter in a saucepan. Mix pepper and
flour, and then pour milk.

4.Cook and whisk until thick and bubbly. Mix cream
cheese until it is even on low heat.

5.Lay vegetables in half quarter casserole dish and put
the sauce over, mix lightly.

6.Put shredded cheese over the top and Bake for about fifteen minutes.

7.Put bread crumbs and leftover butter and dust over on casserole.

8.Bake for twenty-five more min.

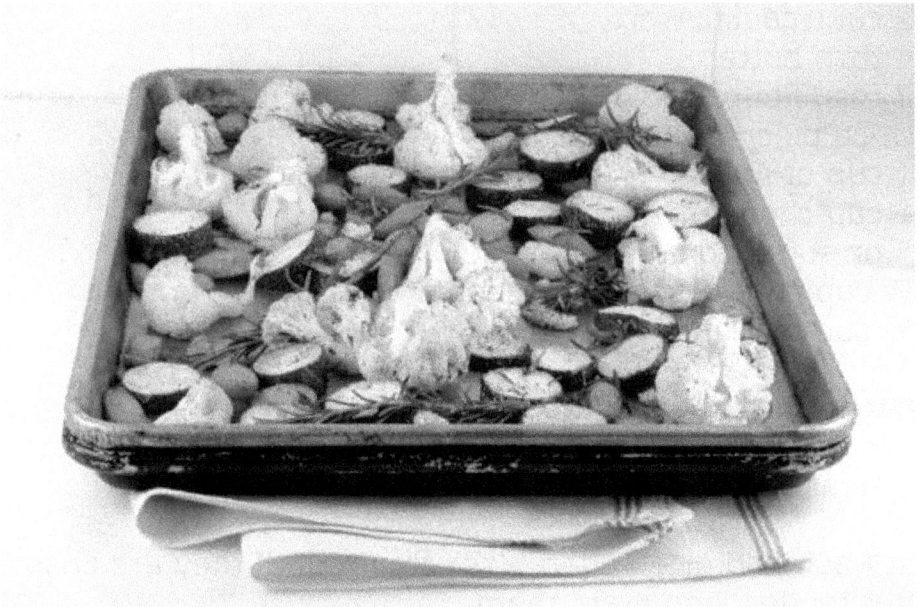

Roasted Fall Vegetables

Preparation time: 20 minutes
Cooking time: 30 minutes
Servings: 8

Ingredients:

1 sliced potato
1 sliced sweet potato
4 sliced and peeled shallots One sliced acorn squash
2 sliced parsnips Two sliced turnips
¼ olive oil Black pepper 6 tbsp butter
4sage leaves
2 tsp Spanish sherry vinegar
One pinch of sea salt

Directions:

1.Heat oven to 400°F prior.

2. Take a large bowl and put vegetables in it.

3.Mix olive oil and season with pepper and salt, if needed. Flip to mix well.

4.Lay vegetables on a baking sheet lined with dish or parchment.

5.Cook, or until vegetables are roasted to sweetness or browned for thirty min.

6.Over medium heat, melt butter in a small saucepan or frying pan.

7.Tear up sage leaves and put them in the saucepan.

8.Remove from heat when the butter gets brown but does not burn. Mix vinegar, salt, and pepper according to taste.

9.Lay each portion of vegetables on its plate. Sprinkle enough of the sage butter to enhance their taste, but don't soak. Enjoy!

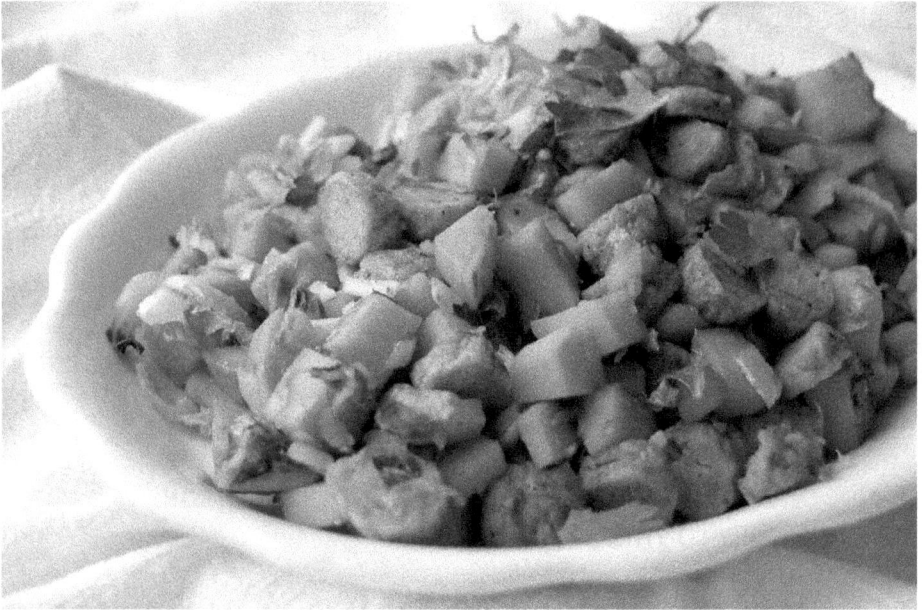

Chickpea Turnip Greens Tacos

Preparation time: 10 minutes
Cooking time: 0 minute
Servings: 12

Ingredients:
6 oz chickpeas
1 minced red onion
1 minced garlic Black pepper
1 tbsp lemon juice
1 tbsp chopped parsley
½ tbsp olive oil
10 oz turnip greens
12 corn tortillas
1 shredded cucumber
2 oz crumbled Feta cheese
¼ tsp sea salt

Directions:
1.Mix garlic, onions, and chickpeas in a large bowl.

2.Spice with salt and pepper, according to taste.

3.Add olive oil, parsley, and lemon juice.

4.Mix until it turns into a chunky paste.

5.Put in thawed turnip greens into this mixture. Mix.

6.Take a warmed corn tortilla (in a skillet or the oven, if you prefer) and put some chickpea turnip greens batter.

7.Dish out with feta cheese and shredded cucumber garnish. Enjoy!

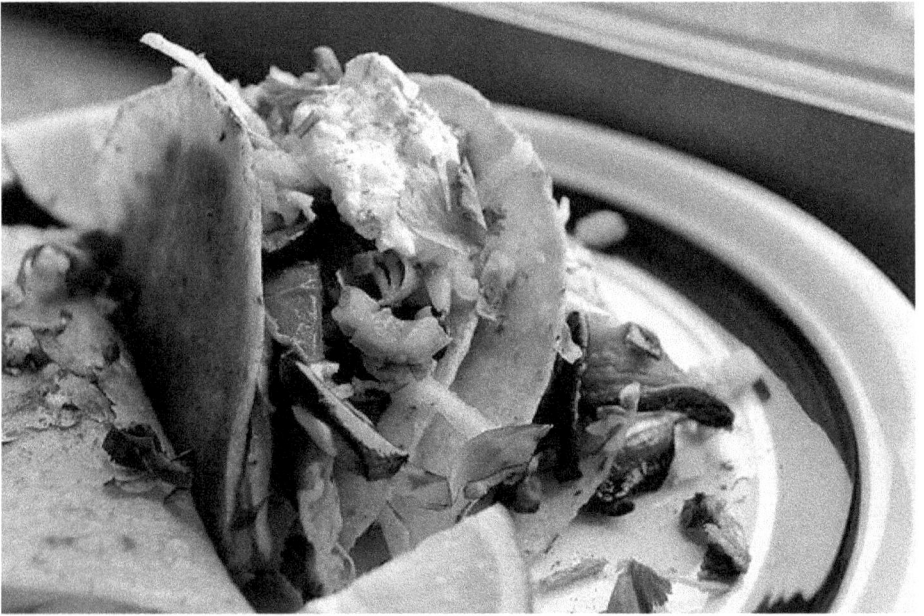

Soy Ginger Roasted Eggplant

Preparation time: 10 minutes
Cooking time: 40 minutes
Servings: 4

Ingredients:

2 eggplants
2 tbsp low sodium soy sauce
½ tsp garlic powder
1 tsp ground ginger
2 tsp olive oil
1/8 tsp pepper

Directions:
1.Heat oven at 400°F prior.

2.Cut the bottom and stem end from the eggplants.
Then slice in half each eggplant lengthwise.

3.Cut deep diagonal lines deep into the eggplant's flesh
about one inch apart, but avoid slicing through the skin.
Turn it over and do the same to make a diamond-
shaped pattern.

4.Take a small bowl and add olive oil, pepper, soy
sauce, ground ginger, and garlic powder. Evenly wrap
the eggplant's flesh side of each half with soy sauce
mixture.

5.Lay the halves' flesh side down onto a foil-lined
baking sheet or parchment.

6.Roast in the oven for thirty to forty min, until the flesh side is browned and caramelized and the skin look collapsed.

7.Once they are cooked through and soft, take it out from the oven, flip the side with the skin side down to cool.

8.Enjoy at room temperature or warm.

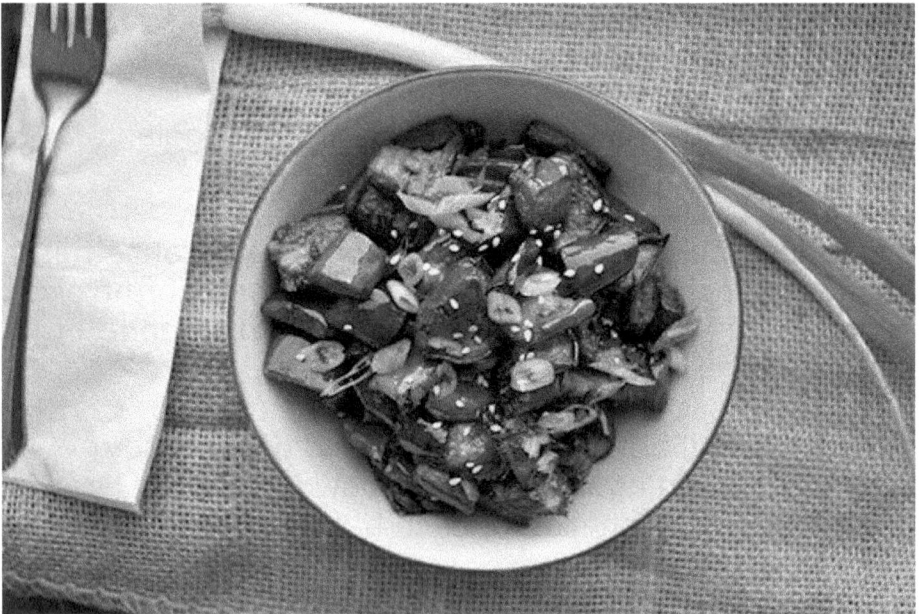

Vegan Shortbread Cookies

Preparation time: 5 minuees
Cooking time: 20 minutes
Servings: 8

Ingredients:

¼ cup of coconut oil
½ cup Powdered sugar
2.5 tbsp yogurt
1 tsp Vanilla extract
½ tsp Cardamom
¼ tsp Salt
1/8 tsp Baking soda
½ cup Whole wheat flour
1 cup flour
1/8 cup chopped cranberries
1/8 cup chopped Apricots
1/8 cup chopped Pecans

Directions:

1.Preheat the oven to 325 degrees.

2.Cream the sugar, coconut oil, and non-dairy yogurt until they become creamy and smooth. Use the hand mixer.

3.Add in the cardamom and vanilla; Mix (for 30-45 seconds).

4.In the flour, now add the salt and baking soda.

5.Mix well using a mixing spoon the ½ cup of the flour mixture in the coconut oil mixture.

6.Do not add flour more than ½ cup at a time to form a soft, fluffy dough. If the mixture becomes too dry, add a tsp. of water. If the mixture becomes too sticky, add a tbsp of flour.

7.Add the nuts and dried fruit to the mixture for this step.

8.Work it thoroughly.

9.Take a 1 to 1 ½ -inch wide log and shape the prepared dough into it. Take a parchment sheet and fold it over the log. Now, freeze for about thirty minutes.

10.Take the log out from the freezer and slice it into ¼ inch slices (or as desired). Take a parchment-lined baking sheet and place the dough on it.

11.For 18-20 minutes, bake it. Adjust the temperature of your oven for the best results. Cool and store! (in an airtight container)

Glazed Green Beans

Preparation time: 5 minutes
Cooking time: 15 minutes
Servings: 6

Ingredients:

12 cups Water
1.5 lb green beans
1 tbsp olive oil
½ tbsp lemon juice
Black pepper to taste
1 tsp Canola oil
1 tbsp Honey
One minced garlic clove
1 tsp Water

Directions:

1.Take a stock-pot. Add water to it and bring it to a boil. Add beans to the water, and cook them until they start turning bright green (for 3 minutes). Be careful not to overcook.

2.Take the beans; rinse and drain with cold water (for about 1 minute). Place them in a bowl and pat them dry thoroughly. Now, set aside.

3.Take separately honey, garlic, 1 tsp. Oil and water; Whisk to make a sauce. Now set aside.

4.Heat one tbsp. Oil in a large pan (medium heat). Add beans to the pan, and stir the beans to coat with oil. Add sauce, continuing to stir, and cook for additional 3 minutes. Finished green beans will be bright green and crisp-tender.

5.Before serving, season the dish with freshly ground black pepper and lemon juice.

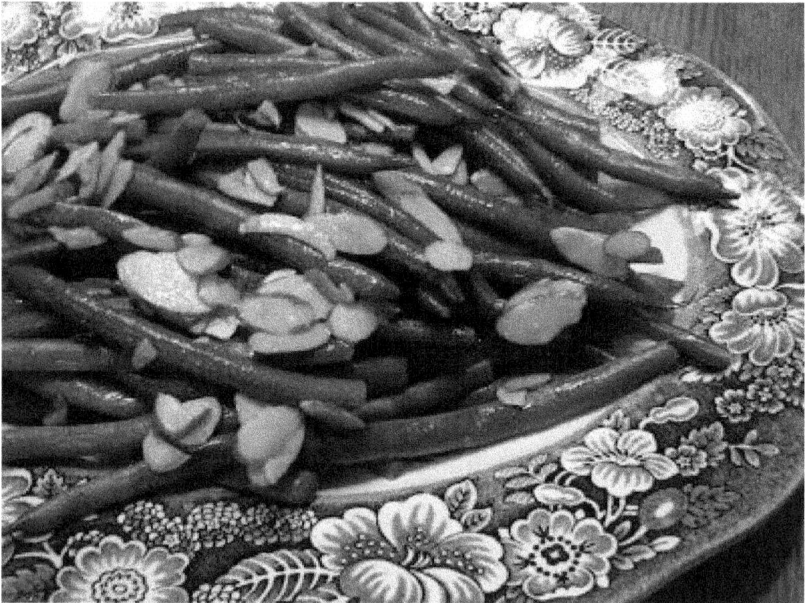

Spicy roasted red pepper hummus

Preparation time: 15 minutes
Cooking time: 60 minutes
Servings: 8

Ingredients:
½ tsp cumin
15 oz garbanzo beans
1.5 tbsp tahini
4 oz roasted red pepper
1 minced garlic clove
½ tsp cayenne pepper
3 tbsp lemon juice
¼ tsp salt
1 tbsp chopped parsley

Directions:

1.Blend all the ingredients in the blender and refrigerator for an hour before serving.

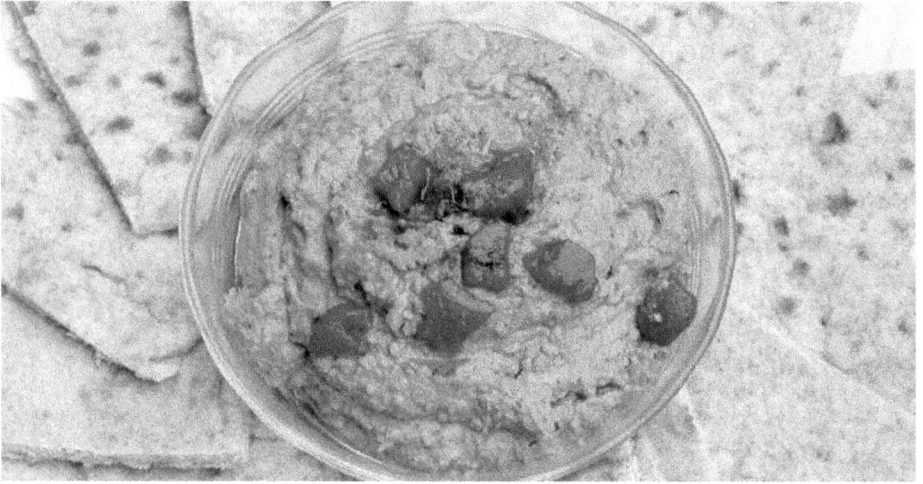

Simple Mediterranean olive oil pasta

Preparation time: 10 minutes
Cooking time: 9 minutes
Servings: 5

Ingredients:

1 lb spaghetti
4 crushed garlic cloves,
½ cup Olive Oil
Salt to taste
12 oz halved grape tomatoes
1 cup chopped parsley
Red pepper flakes crushed
3 chopped scallions
6 oz marinated artichoke hearts
1 tsp black pepper
¼ cup halved pitted olives
12 torn basil leaves
¼ cup crumbled feta cheese
Zest of one lemon

Directions:

1.Cook pasta according to the instructions given on the box.

2.Sauté garlic and salt in heated olive oil over medium flame.

3.Add tomatoes, scallions, and parsley. Cook for one minute.

4.Pour the garlic sauce over the cooked and drained pasta.

5.Sprinkle pepper and leftover ingredients and toss well.

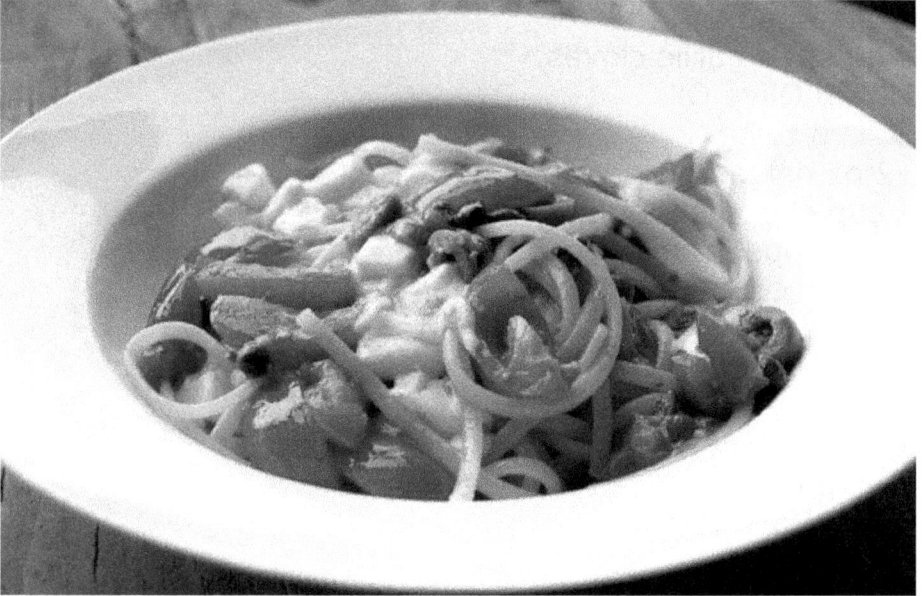

Roasted vegetable barley

Preparation time: 10 minutes
Cooking time: 40 minutes
Servings: 6

Ingredients:

1 cup pearl barley
2 diced zucchini squash water
1diced bell pepper (red and yellow)
2 oz chopped parsley
Salt to taste
1 diced red onion black pepper to taste
¾ tsp smoked paprika
2 tsp harissa spice Olive oil
1 minced garlic clove
2 chopped scallions
Feta cheese
2 tbsp lemon juice
Toasted pine nuts

Directions:

1.Boil barley in water for 45 minutes.

2.In a bowl, mix veggies, salt, harissa spice, paprika, pepper, and oil.

3.Roast in a preheated oven at 425 degrees for 25 minutes.

4.Transfer the roasted veggies, cooked barley, scallions, parsley, garlic, lemon juice, and oil in a large bowl and mix to coat well.

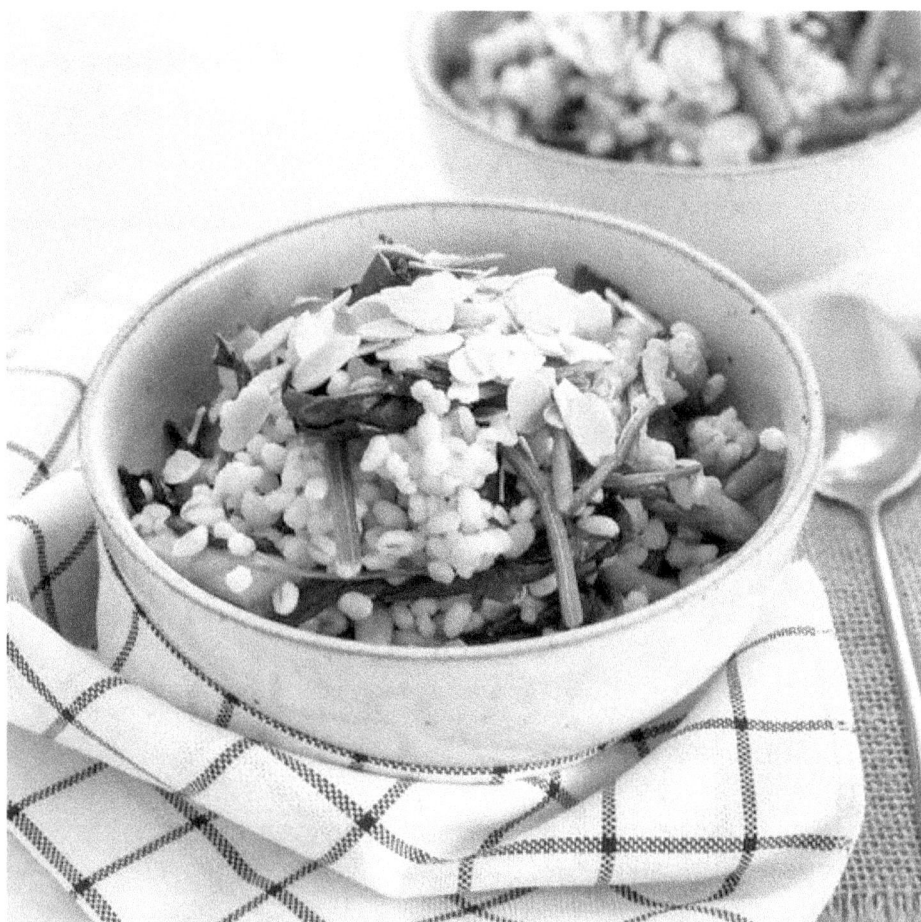

Moroccan couscous

Preparation time: 10 minutes
Cooking time: 10 minutes
Servings: 5

Ingredients:

2 cups couscous
4 cups flavorful stock
2 tbsp olive oil
1 tsp salt
1/2 tsp black pepper

Directions:

1.Boil stock, oil, salt, and pepper in the pot.

2.Transfer the potting mixture to a bowl, add couscous and toss.

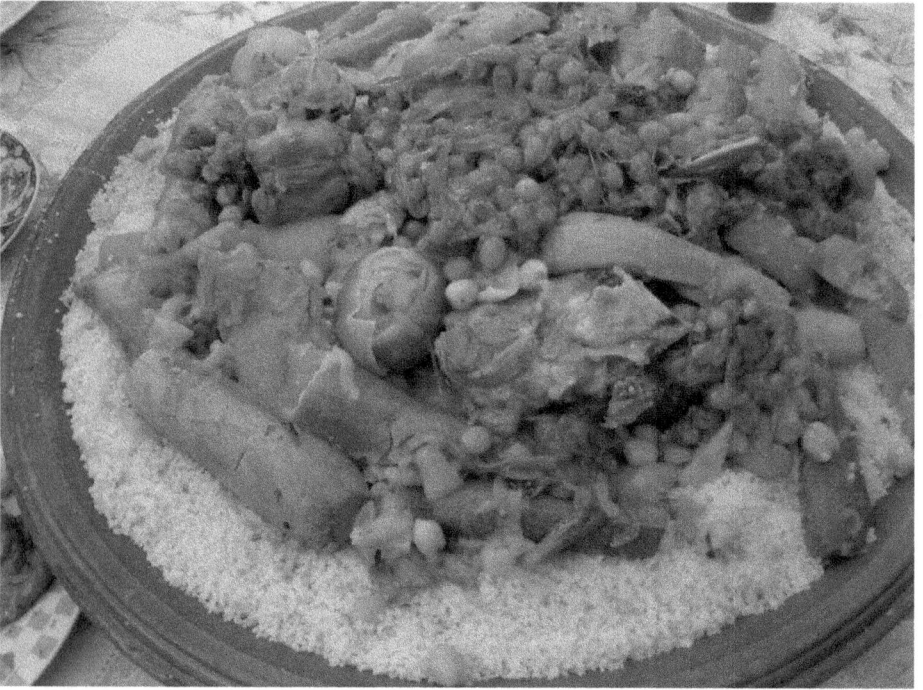

Simple tuna pasta

Preparation time: 5 minutes
Cooking time: 10 minutes
Servings: 2

Ingredients:

2 tbsp olive oil
2 minced cloves garlic
5 oz tuna
1 tsp lemon juice
1 tbsp chopped parsley
Salt to taste
Black pepper to taste
4 oz uncooked pasta

Directions:

1.Cook pasta accordingly in boiling water for seven minutes.

2.Sauté garlic in heated oil for half a minute over medium flame.

3.Add tuna, parsley, and lemon juice. Cook for another minute.

4.Add three spoons of pasta water and mix well.

5.Mix drained pasta and toss well.

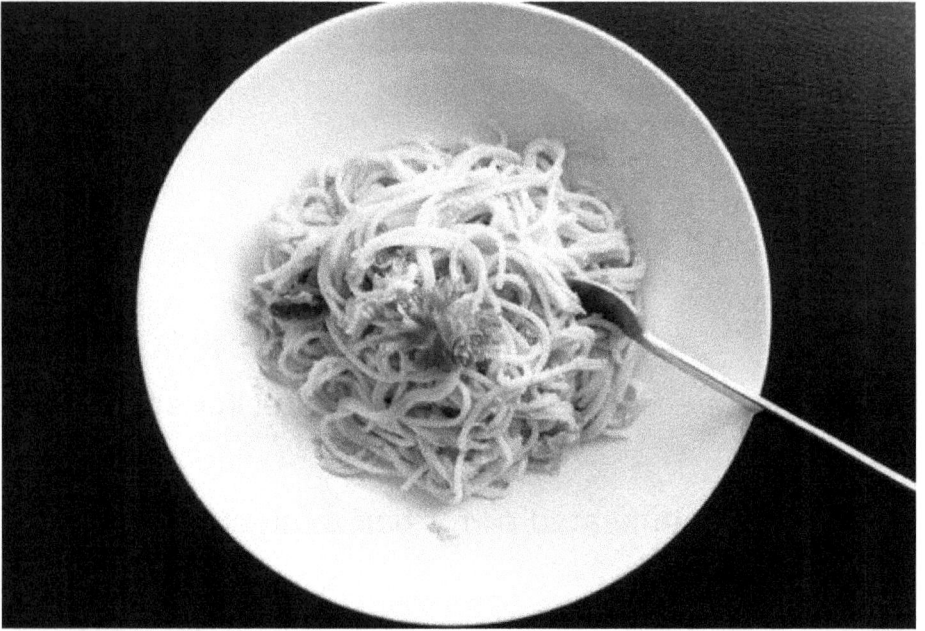

Mushroom barley soup

Preparation time: 15 minutes
Cooking time: 60 minutes
Servings: 4

Ingredients:

Olive oil
16 oz sliced Bella mushrooms Kosher
salt to taste
1 chopped yellow onion,
4 minced garlic cloves
2 chopped celery stalks
1 diced carrot
8 oz chopped white mushrooms
½ cup crushed tomatoes
Black pepper to taste
1 tsp coriander
½ tsp smoked paprika
½ tsp cumin 6 cups broth
1 cup pearl barley
½ cup chopped parsley

Directions:

1.Cook mushrooms in heated olive oil over a high flame in a Dutch oven for seven minutes and keep it aside.

2.Sauté onions, carrots, white mushrooms, and celery in the same pan with more olive oil for five minutes over medium flame. Sprinkle pepper and salt.

3.Stir in tomatoes and spices. Cook for five more minutes.

4.Mix barley and broth and boil for five minutes.

5.Simmer it for 45 minutes over low flame.

6.Add cooked mushrooms and cook for few more minutes.

7.Sprinkle parsley and serve.

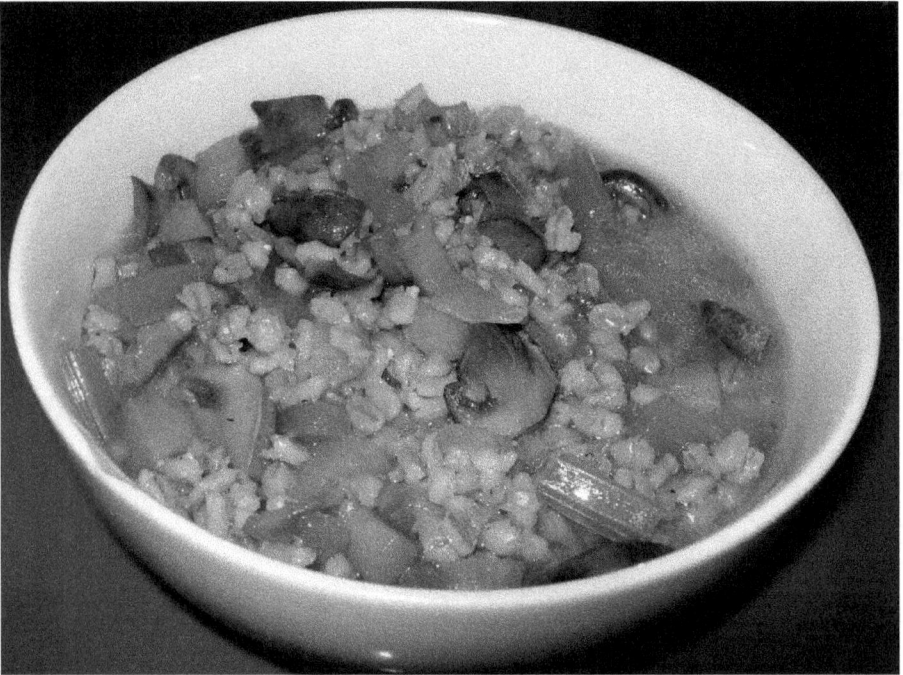

Mediterranean couscous salad

Preparation time: 15 minutes
Cooking time: 10 minutes
Servings: 6

Ingredients:

Lemon-Dill Vinaigrette
1 tbsp lemon juice
1/3 cup olive oil
1 tsp dill
1.5 minced garlic cloves
Salt to taste
Black pepper to taste
Israeli Couscous
2 cups Pearl Couscous
3 oz mozzarella cheese
Water
Olive oil
2 cups grape tomatoes
1/2 chopped English cucumber
1/3 cup chopped red onions
15 oz chickpeas
½ cup Kalamata olives
14 oz chopped artichoke hearts 18 chopped basil leaves

Directions:

1.Mix all the ingredients of vinaigrette in a container and set aside. The lemon dill vinaigrette is ready.

2.Cook couscous in heated olive oil over medium flame.

3.Pour boiling water about three cups and cook until couscous Is cooked.

4.Combine all the leftover ingredients in a bowl except mozzarella.

5.Mix couscous with the ingredients.

6.Pour vinaigrette and toss well.

7.Sprinkle mozzarella and serve.

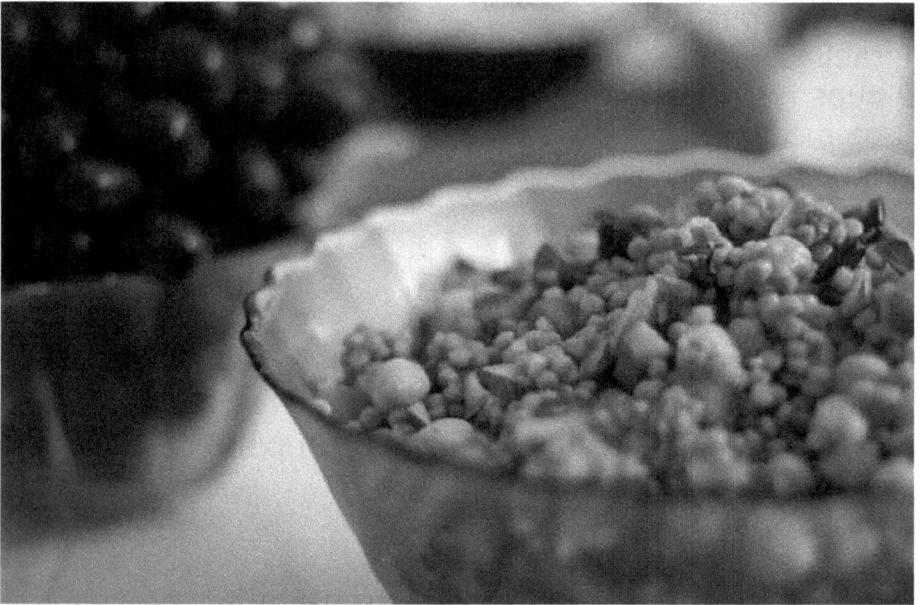

Italian minestrone

Preparation time: 10 minutes
Cooking time: 25 minutes
Servings: 6

Ingredients:
1 tbsp olive oil
1 cup diced celery
1 cup diced yellow onion
1 cup diced carrots
1 cup diced yellow squash
1 cup diced zucchini
1 tbsp minced garlic
2 tbsp tomato paste
4 cups vegetable broth
28 oz diced tomatoes
1 cup dried pasta
1 tsp salt One bay leaf
2rosemary sprigs
1 tsp chopped dried oregano
1 cup green beans
15 oz red beans Black pepper to taste
2 tsp chopped parsley

Directions:

1.Sauté onions. Carrots and celery in heated olive oil in a Dutch oven over high flame for five minutes.

2.Mix squash and zucchini and cook for two more minutes.

3.Stir in garlic and tomato paste and cook.

4.Pour vegetable stock. Add tomatoes, salt, bay leaf, rosemary, and oregano, and toss well.

5.Let it boil and simmer over medium flame.

6.Mix pasta and red beans and cook for ten minutes.

7.Add greens beans and cook for three minutes.

8.Adjust the consistency of the soup b adding the stock.

9.Adjust the taste and toss well before serving.

Lebanese rice with vermicelli

Preparation time: 15 minutes
Cooking time: 20 minutes
Servings: 6

Ingredients:

Salt to taste
2 cups long-grain rice
1 cup broken vermicelli Water
2.5 tbsp olive oil
½ cup toasted pine nuts

Directions:

1.Soak rice in water for 30 minutes.

2.Cook vermicelli in heated olive oil over a high flame until it turned brown.

3.Mix drained rice and mix. Sprinkle salt and continue stirring to mix them well.

4.Add water and boil it to concentrate the mixture.

5.Reduce the heat, cover, and cook for 21 minutes over low flame.

6.Serve and enjoy it.

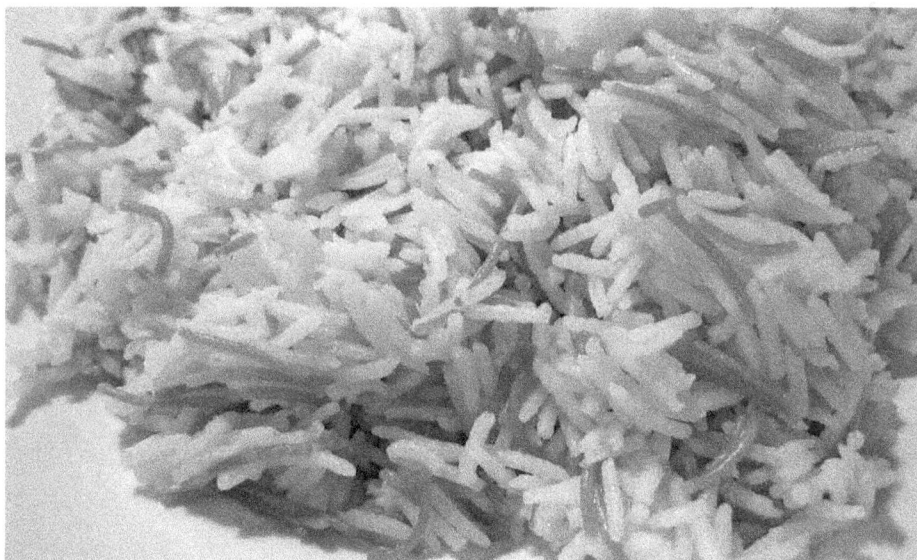

Penne with Tomato, Basil and Parmesan Cheese

Preparation time: 5 minutes
Cooking time: 20 minutes
Servings: 4

Ingredients:
Twelve cups water
Three cups dry penne
3 tbsp olive oil extra virgin
12 oz grape tomatoes
2 tbsp minced garlic
One cup chopped basil
4 tbsp shredded parmesan cheese

Directions:

1.Boil a large pot of water. Add pasta and cook for twelve minutes, or until al dente. Occasionally stir it. Drain the cooked pasta using a filter and put it aside.

2.Add and heat two tbsp of olive oil to a medium-sized saucepan over medium-high heat. Once it is hot, add and sauté tomatoes until they are soft for almost two minutes.

3.Put garlic and cook for an extra minute.

4.Add pasta and also leftover tbsp of olive oil to the saucepan, and fry for 1 min.

5.Add three by four cups of basil and toss the pan until it is evenly distributed.

6. Adorn it with leftover parmesan cheese and chopped basil, and serve right away.

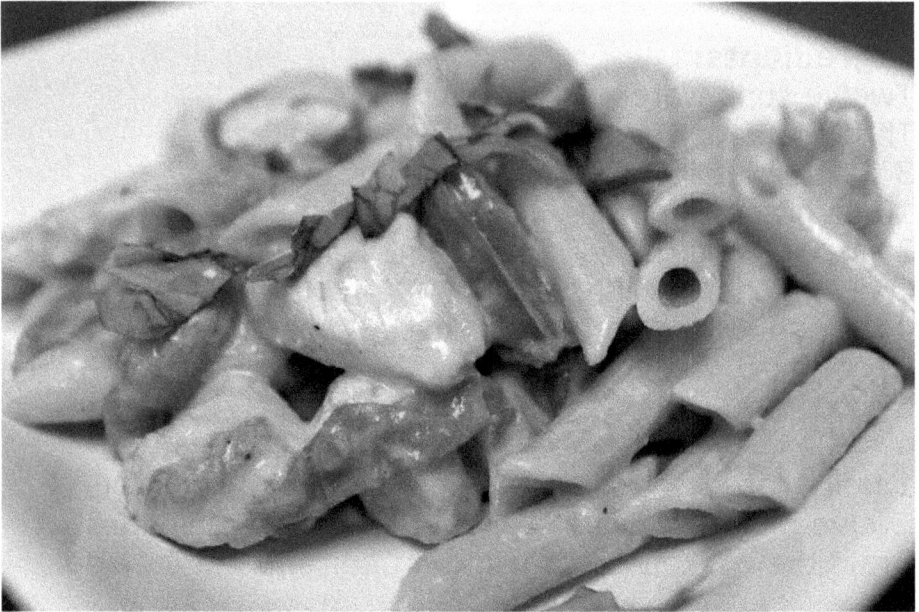

Delightful Bulgur Pilaf

Preparation time: 15 minutes
Cooking time: 10 minutes
Servings: 5

Ingredients:

1 cup of water
1 chopped tomato
1 cup bulgur wheat
1 cup corn kernels
¼ cup dill

Directions:

1.Take a tomato, bulgur, and water and boil it in a saucepan over high heat.

2.Put in dill and corn and reduce the heat.

3.Fry for almost five minutes frequently.

4.If required and one by the fourth cup, add more water until the bulgur is not soggy but tender.

5.Until the water is absorbed, Cook it. It turns into a pilaf, like rice cooked with other ingredients.

6.Remove from the stove. Wrap and let stand for five to seven minutes.

7.Serve with a green salad for lunch or as a side dish to seafood or meat for dinner. Enjoy!

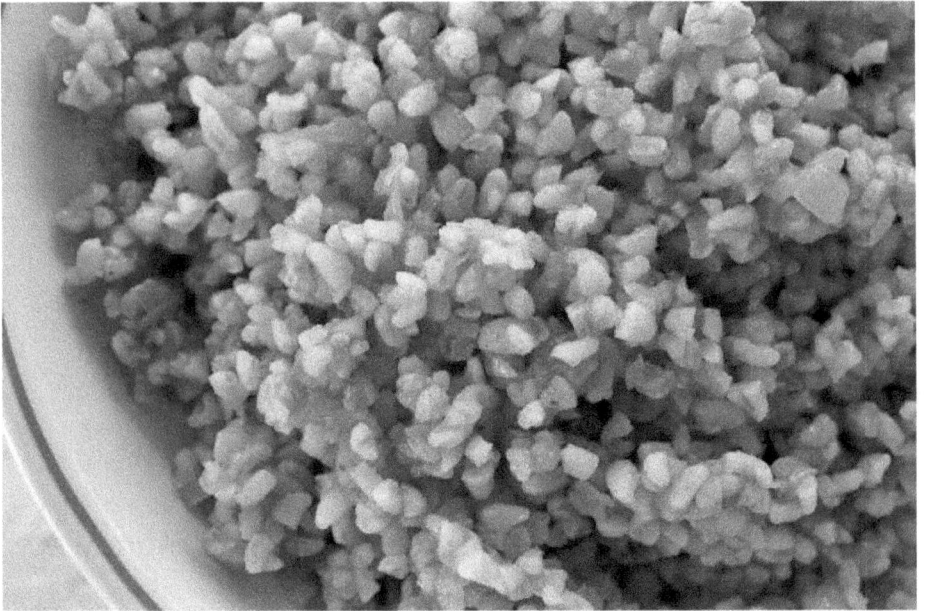

Corn Pudding

Preparation time: 10 minutes
Cooking time: 40 minutes
Servings: 6

Ingredients:
Butter
2 tbsp all-purpose flour
½ tsp baking soda
3 eggs
¾ cup of rice milk
3 tbsp melted butter
2 tbsp light sour cream
2 tbsp granulated sugar
2cups corn kernels

Directions:
1.Heat the oven before 350°F.

2.Lightly lubricate with butter an eight by an eight-inch baking dish, and put it aside.

3.Take a small bowl, mix flour and baking soda substitute, and put it aside.

4.Take a medium-sized bowl and beat together sugar, butter, sour cream, eggs, and rice milk.

5.Blend the egg mixture into the flour mixture until even.

6.Mix the corn to the mixture and stir until even.

7.Spoon this mixture in the baking dish and bake until the pudding is set, for almost forty minutes.

8.Let it cool for fifteen minutes and serve warm.

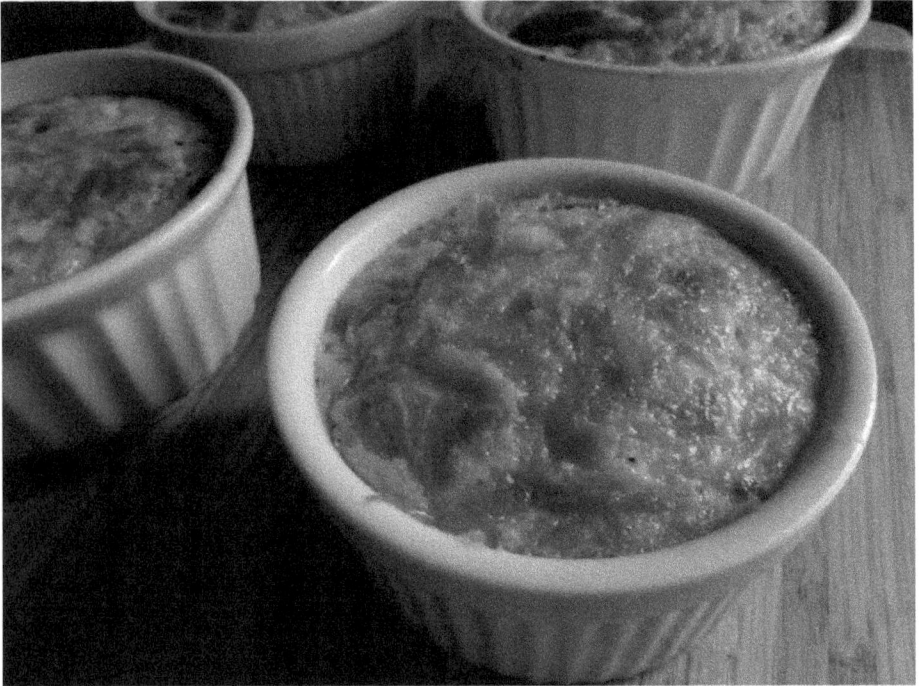

Egg White Frittata with Penne

Preparation time: 15 minutes
Cooking time: 30 minutes
Servings: 4-5

Ingredients:

6 egg whites
¼ cup of rice milk
1 tbsp chopped parsley
1 tbsp chopped thyme
1 tsp chopped chives
Black pepper to taste
2 tbsp olive oil
¼ chopped sweet onion
1 tsp minced garlic
½ cup chopped red bell pepper (boiled)
2 cups cooked penne

Directions:

1.Heat the oven at 350°F prior.

2.Whisk egg whites, chives, parsley, rice milk thyme, and pepper in a large bowl.

3.Warm olive oil over medium heat in an ovenproof frying pan.

4.Fry the garlic, red pepper, and onion for four min until they are soft.

5.Add the cooked penne to the frying pan using a spatula to pour the pasta evenly.

6.Cover the pasta with egg mixture and shake the pan, distribute it evenly.

7.Set the frittata's bottom, leave the frying pan on the heat for one minute, and then move the pan to the oven.

8.Bake it for twenty-five min until it is golden brown and set.

9. Take it out from the oven and dish it up immediately.

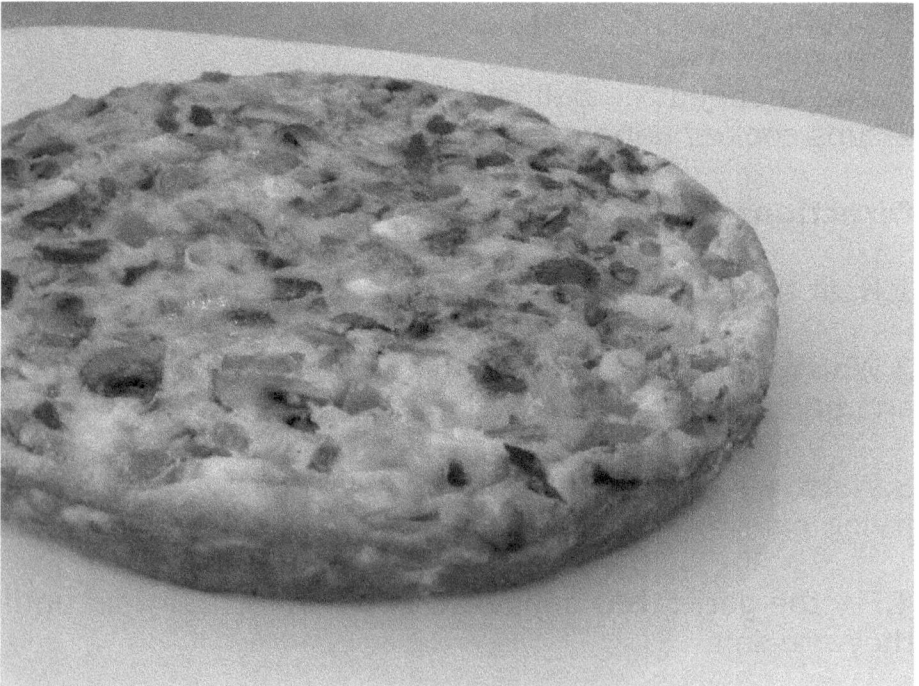

Delicious White Bean Hummus

Preparation time: 10 minutes
Cooking time: 25 minutes
Serves:16

Ingredients:

Roasted Tomatoes as needed
1 head of garlic
30 ounce cooked cannellini beans
1 tbsp lemon juice
1/2 tsp salt

Directions:

1.Set the oven to 400 degrees F and let it preheat meanwhile remove the tip of the garlic head and loose papery coating.

2.Get a 6 ounce custard cup and add garlic. Drizzle with 1 tsp of oil and then cover it with foil.

3.Place your custard into the heated oven and bake for 25 minutes until the garlic head is soft. When it is done uncover the custard cup let it cool and squeeze the garlic.

4.Place the garlic into a food processor and add the cannellini beans lemon juice oil and salt. Pulse until well blended.

5.Tip the hummus into the bowl and drizzle with olive oil. Add roasted tomatoes and serve with some vegetables.

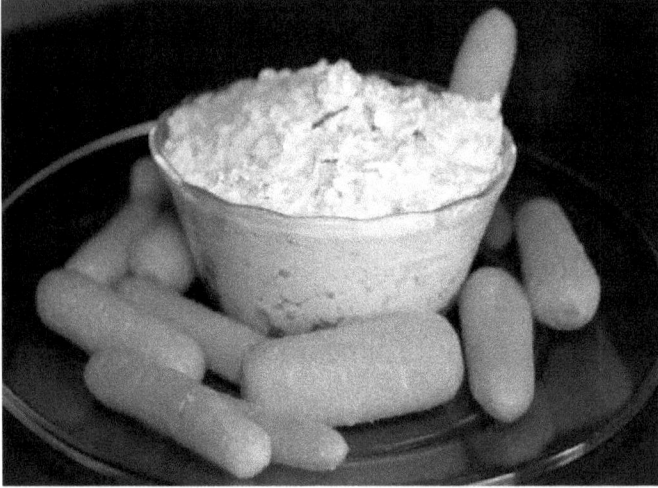

Garlic with Escarole

Preparation time: 5 minutes
Cooking time: 7 minutes
Serves:4

Ingredients:

1 and 1/2 tsp of garlic
1 head of escarole leaves torn
1/8 tsp red pepper flakes
1 and 1/2 tbsp olive oil
1 tsp salt

Directions:

1.Place a medium skillet pan over medium high heat. Add garlic and cook for a couple of minutes until nicely golden brown. Stir in the red pepper flakes and add the escarole in batches. Season with salt and toss until it is well incorporated.

2.Cook this for 5 minutes until the escarole leaves wilt. Serve immediately.

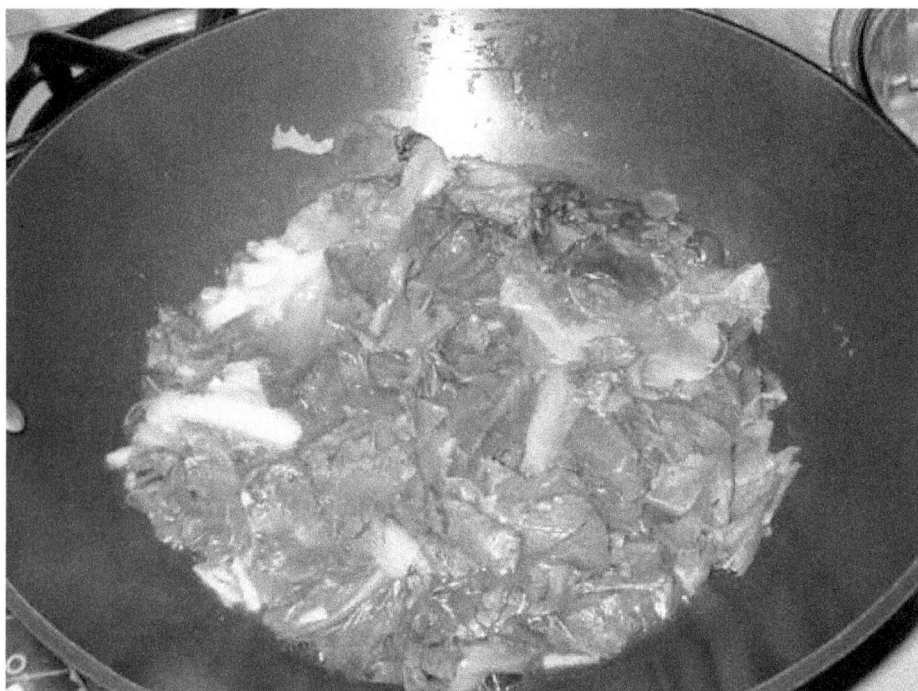

Cheddar Potato Crisps

Preparation Time: 10 minutes
Cooking Time: 0 minutes
Servings: 4

Ingredients:
1 cup Greek yogurt (unsweetened)
1/2 cup grated cheddar cheese
6 red potatoes, thinly sliced
1/2 cup chives
3 slices ham
Cooking oil or spray as required Salt and black pepper
to taste

Directions:

1.Take the potatoes; sprinkle with salt and black pepper.

2.Cover and place in the refrigerator for 30 minutes.

3.Heat a grill at medium temperature setting.

4.Spray the potato slices with cooking oil, place over a baking sheet and grill for about 2 minutes.

5.Flip and grill for 2 more minutes. Add the ham slices to the baking sheet and grill for one minute.

6.Add the potato and ham in a serving bowl. Top with the chives, yogurt and grated cheese as desired.

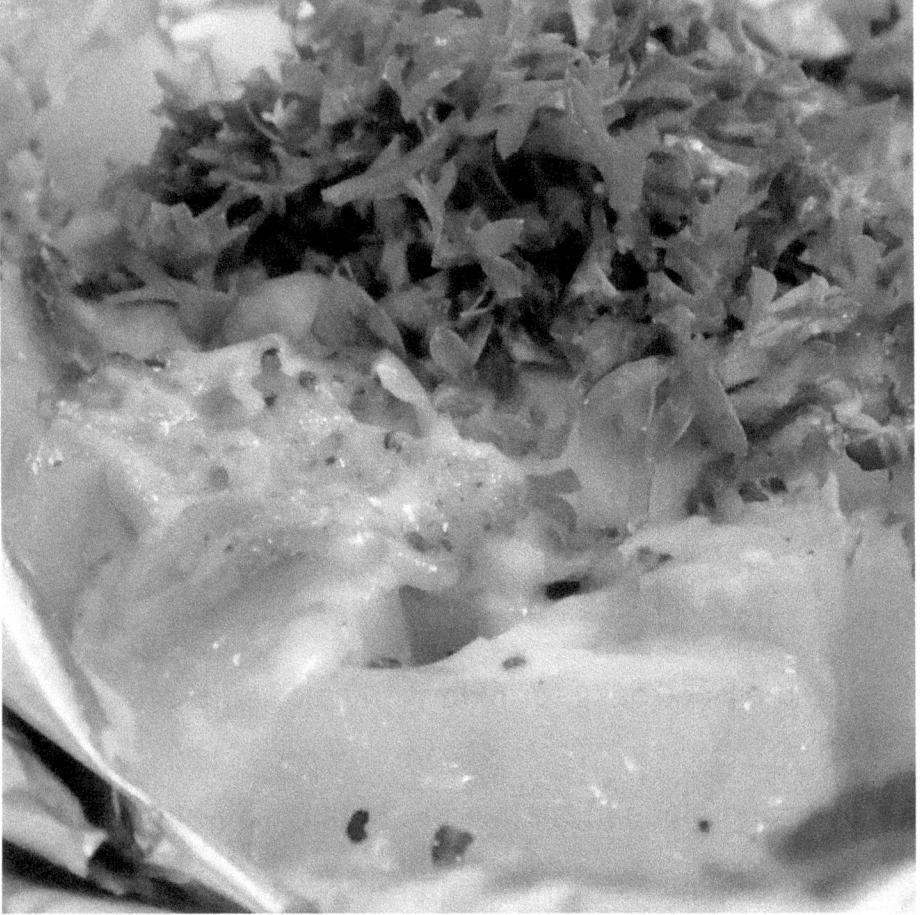

Healthy Coconut Blueberry Balls

Preparation Time: 10 minutes

Cooking Time: 10 minutes

Servings: 12

Ingredients:

¼ cup flaked coconut
¼ cup blueberries
½ tsp. vanilla
¼ cup honey
½ cup creamy almond butter
¼ tsp. cinnamon
1 ½ tbsp. chia seeds
¼ cup flaxseed meal
1 cup rolled oats, gluten-free

Directions:

1. In a large bowl, add oats, cinnamon, chia seeds, and flaxseed meal and mix well.

2. Add almond butter in microwave-safe bowl and microwave for 30 seconds. Stir until smooth.

3. Add vanilla and honey in melted almond butter and stir well.

4. Pour almond butter mixture over oat mixture and stir to combine.

5. Add coconut and blueberries and stir well.

6.Make small balls from oat mixture and place onto the baking tray and place in the refrigerator for 1 hour.

7.Serve and enjoy.

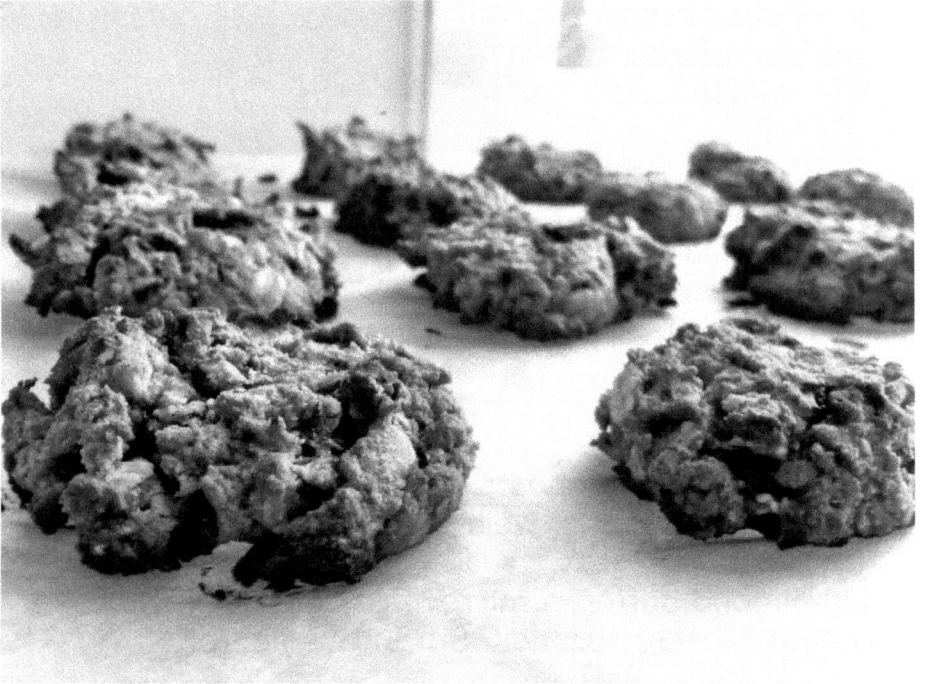

Crunchy Roasted Chickpeas

Preparation Time: 10 minutes

Cooking Time: 25 minutes

Servings: 4

Ingredients:
15 oz can chickpeas, drained, rinsed and pat dry
¼ tsp. paprika
1 tbsp. olive oil
¼ tsp. pepper Pinch of salt

Directions:

1.Preheat the oven to 450°F.

2.Spray a baking tray with cooking spray and set aside.

3.In a large bowl, toss chickpeas with olive oil and spread chickpeas onto the prepared baking tray.

4.Roast chickpeas in preheated oven for 25 minutes. Shake after every 10 minutes.

5.Once chickpeas are done then immediately toss with paprika, pepper, and salt.

6.Serve and enjoy.

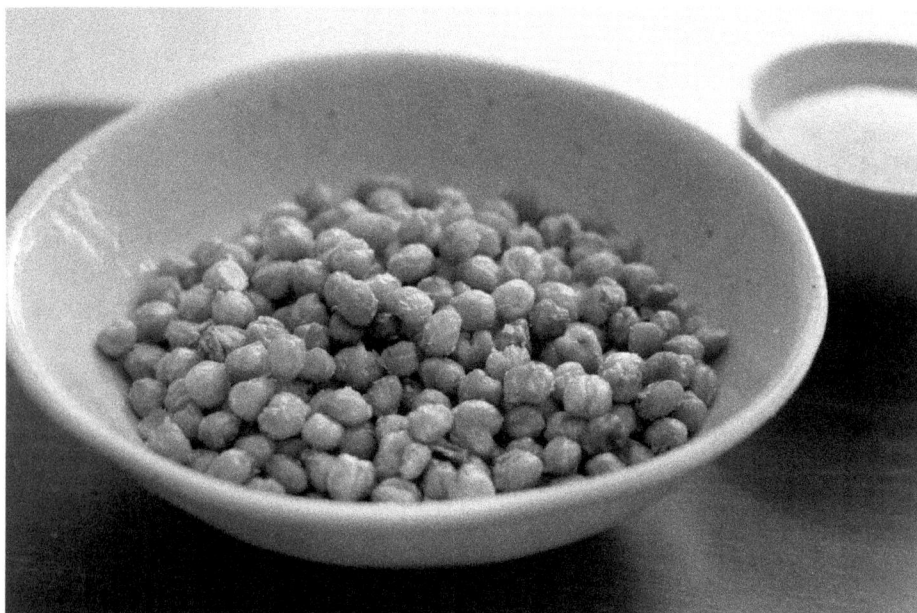

Tasty Zucchini Chips

Preparation Time: 10 minutes
Cooking Time: 15 minutes
Servings: 8

Ingredients:

2 medium zucchini, sliced 4mm thick
½ tsp. paprika
¼ tsp. garlic powder
¾ cup parmesan cheese, grated
4 tbsp. olive oil
¼ tsp. pepper Pinch of salt

Directions:

1.Preheat the oven to 375°F.

2.Spray a baking tray with cooking spray and set aside.

3.In a bowl, combine the oil, garlic powder, paprika, pepper, and salt.

4.Add sliced zucchini and toss to coat.

5.Arrange zucchini slices onto the prepared baking tray and sprinkle grated cheese on top.

6.Bake in preheated oven for 15 minutes or until lightly golden brown.

7.Serve and enjoy.

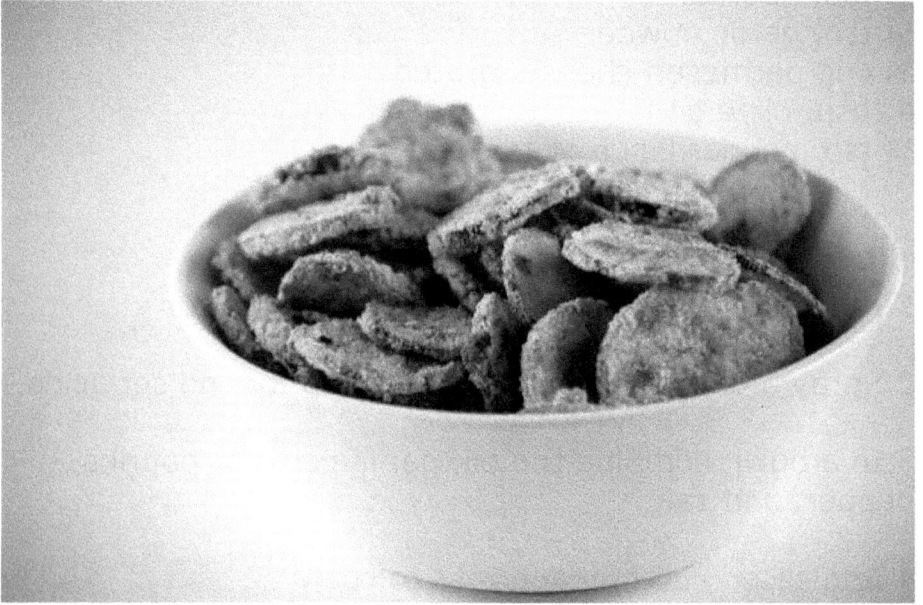

Roasted Green Beans

Preparation Time: 10 minutes
Cooking Time: 15 minutes
Servings: 4

Ingredients:

1 lb green beans
4 tbsp. parmesan cheese
2 tbsp. olive oil
¼ tsp. garlic powder
Pinch of salt

Directions:

1. Preheat the oven to 400°F.

2. Add green beans in a large bowl.

3. Add remaining ingredients on top of green beans and toss to coat.

4. Spread green beans onto the baking tray and roast in preheated oven for 15 minutes. Stir halfway through.

5. Serve and enjoy.

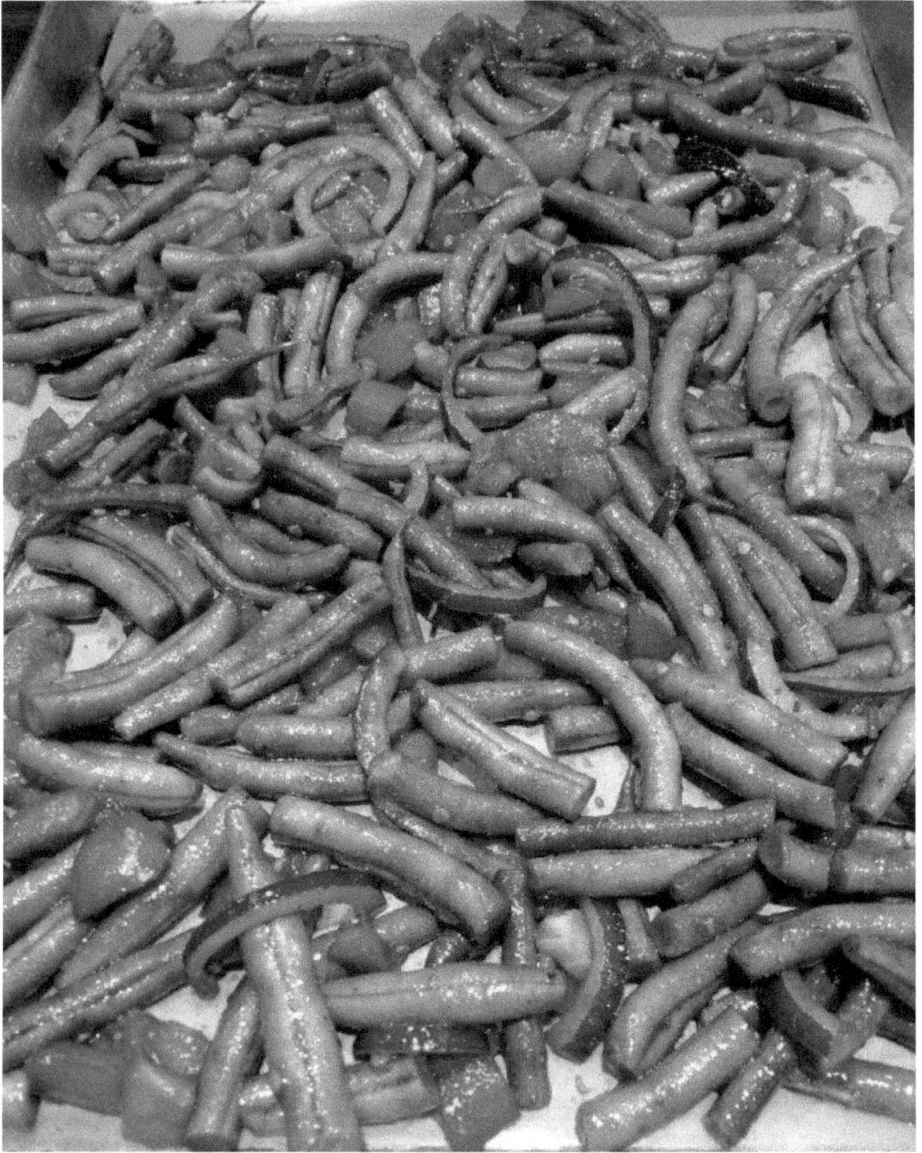

Savory Pistachio Balls

Preparation Time: 10 minutes
Cooking Time: 5 minutes
Servings: 16

Ingredients:

½ cup pistachios, unsalted
1 cup dates, pitted
½ tsp. ground fennel seeds
½ cup raisins
Pinch of pepper

Directions:

1.Add all ingredients into the food processor and process until well combined.

2.Make small balls and place onto the baking tray and place in the refrigerator for 1 hour.

3.Serve and enjoy.

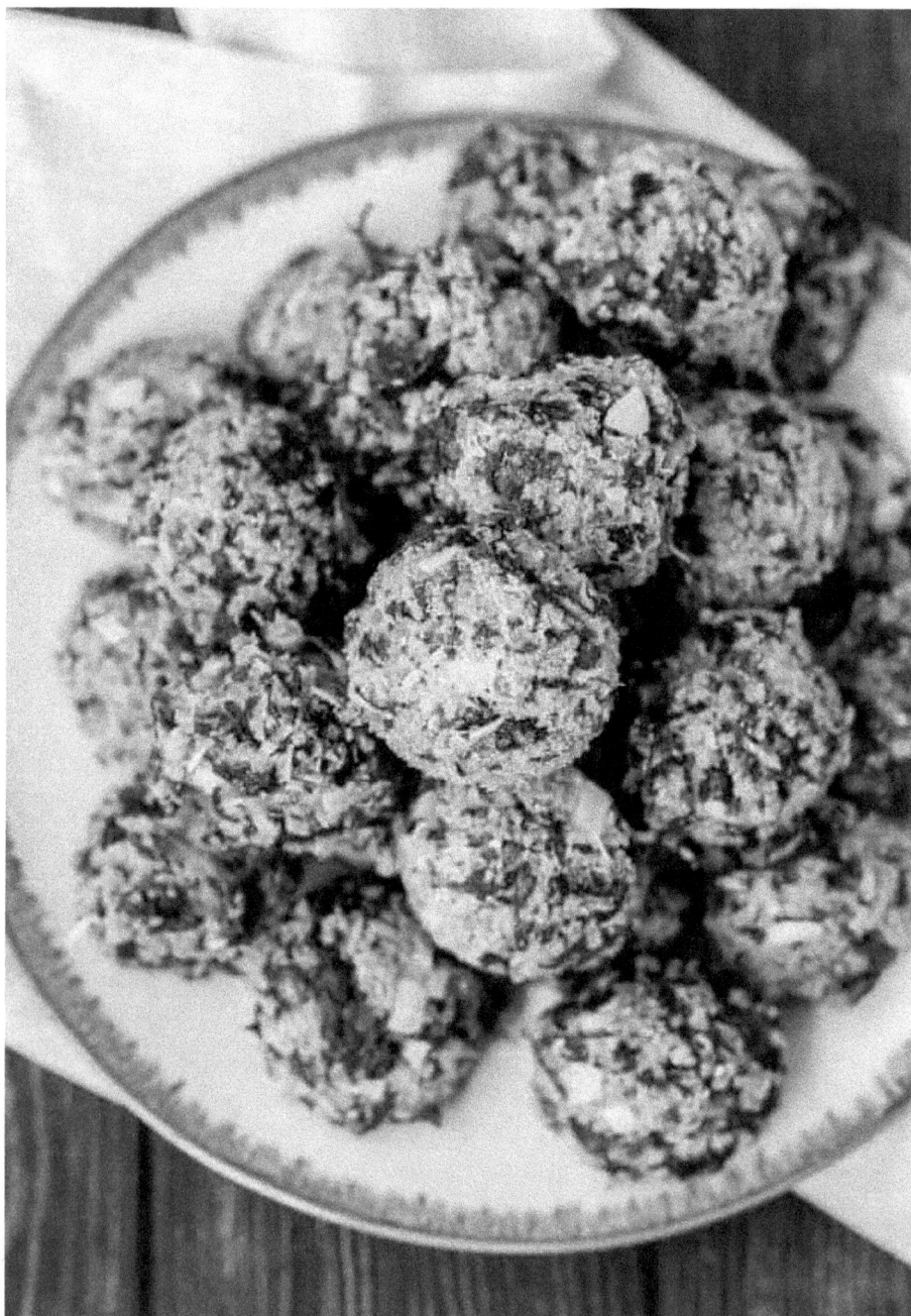

Roasted Almonds

Preparation Time: 10 minutes
Cooking Time: 20 minutes
Servings: 12

Ingredients:
2 ½ cups almonds
¼ tsp. cayenne
¼ tsp. ground coriander
¼ tsp. cumin
¼ tsp. chili powder
1 tbsp. fresh rosemary, chopped
1 tbsp. olive oil
2 ½ tbsp. maple syrup
Pinch of salt

Directions:

1.Preheat the oven to 325°F.

2.Spray a baking tray with cooking spray and set aside.

3.In a mixing bowl, whisk together oil, cayenne, coriander, cumin, chili powder, rosemary, maple syrup, and salt.

4.Add almond and stir to coat.

5.Spread almonds onto the prepared baking tray.

6.Roast almonds in preheated oven for 20 minutes. Stir halfway through.

7.Serve and enjoy.

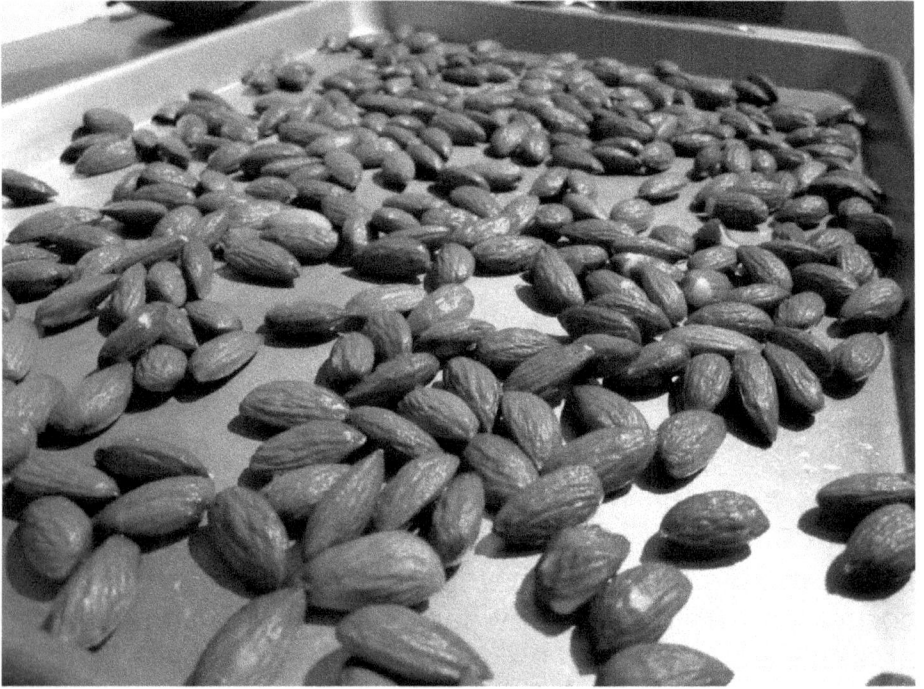

Banana Strawberry Popsicles

Preparation Time: 5 minutes

Cooking Time: 0 minutes

Servings: 8

Ingredients:

½ cup Greek yogurt
1 banana, peeled and sliced
1 ¼ cup fresh strawberries
¼ cup of water

Directions:

1.Add all ingredients into the blender and blend until smooth.

2.Pour blended mixture into the popsicles molds and place in the refrigerator for 4 hours or until set.

3.Serve and enjoy.

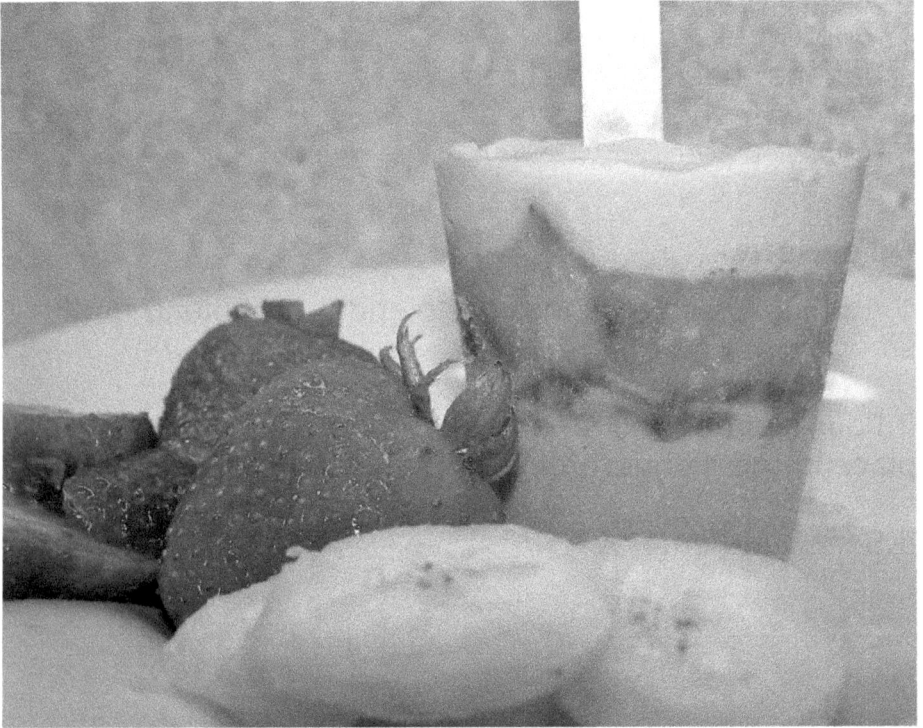

Chocolate Matcha Balls

Preparation Time: 10 minutes
Cooking Time: 5 minutes
Servings: 15

Ingredients:

2 tbsp. unsweetened cocoa powder
3 tbsp. oats, gluten-free
½ cup pine nuts
½ cup almonds
1 cup dates, pitted
2 tbsp. matcha powder

Directions:

1.Add oats, pine nuts, almonds, and dates into a food processor and process until well combined.

2.Place matcha powder in a small dish.

3.Make small balls from mixture and coat with matcha powder.

4.Enjoy or store in refrigerator until ready to eat.

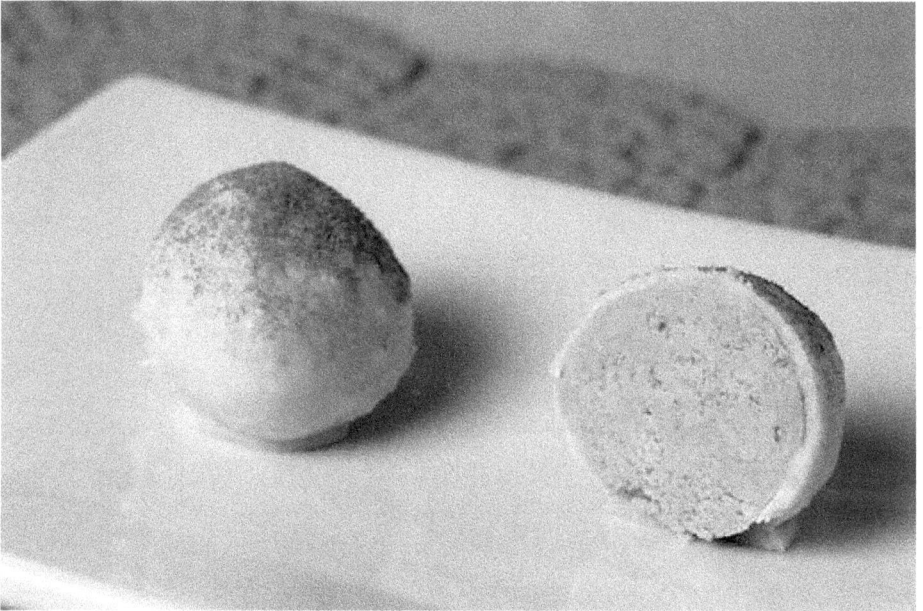

Chia Almond Butter Pudding

Preparation Time: 5 minutes

Cooking Time: 5 minutes

Servings: 1

Ingredients:

¼ cup chia seeds
1 cup unsweetened almond milk
1 ½ tbsp. maple syrup
2 ½ tbsp. almond butter

Directions:

1.Add almond milk, maple syrup, and almond butter in a bowl and stir well.

2.Add chia seeds and stir to mix.

3.Pour pudding mixture into the Mason jar and place in the refrigerator for overnight.

4.Serve and enjoy.

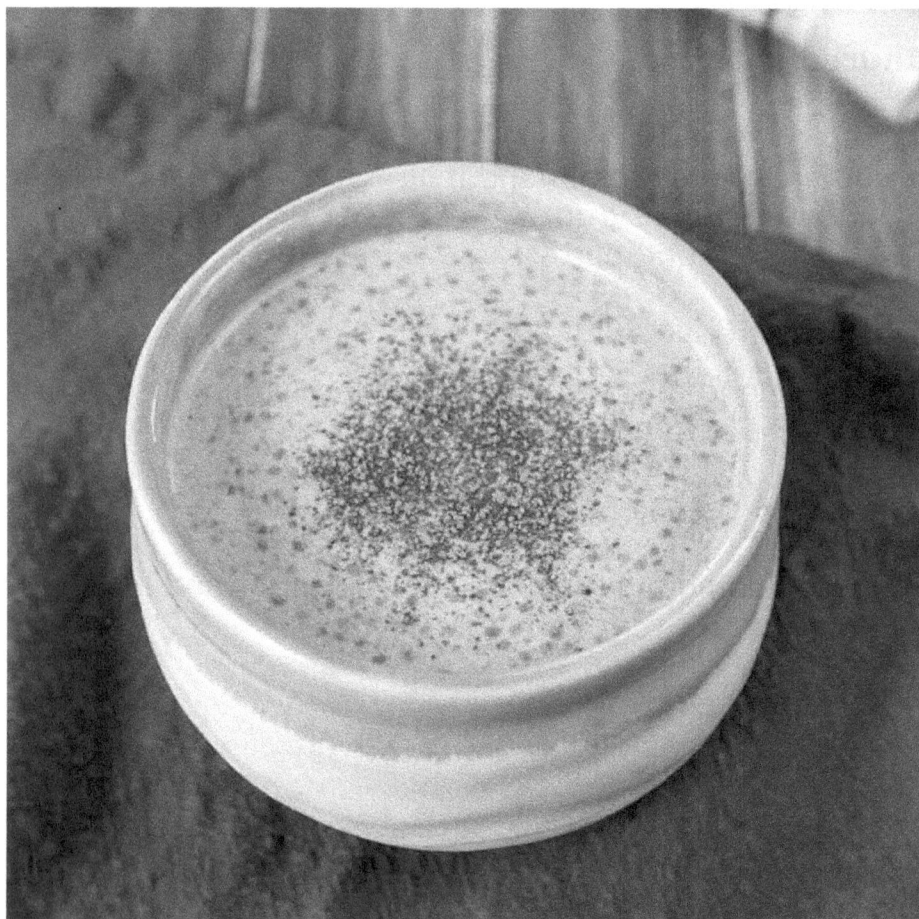

Refreshing Strawberry Popsicles

Preparation Time: 5 minutes

Cooking Time: 5 minutes

Servings: 8

Ingredients:
½ cup almond milk
2 ½ cup fresh strawberries

Directions:

1.Add strawberries and almond milk into the blender and blend until smooth.

2.Pour strawberry mixture into popsicles molds and place in the refrigerator for 4 hours or until set.

3.Serve and enjoy.

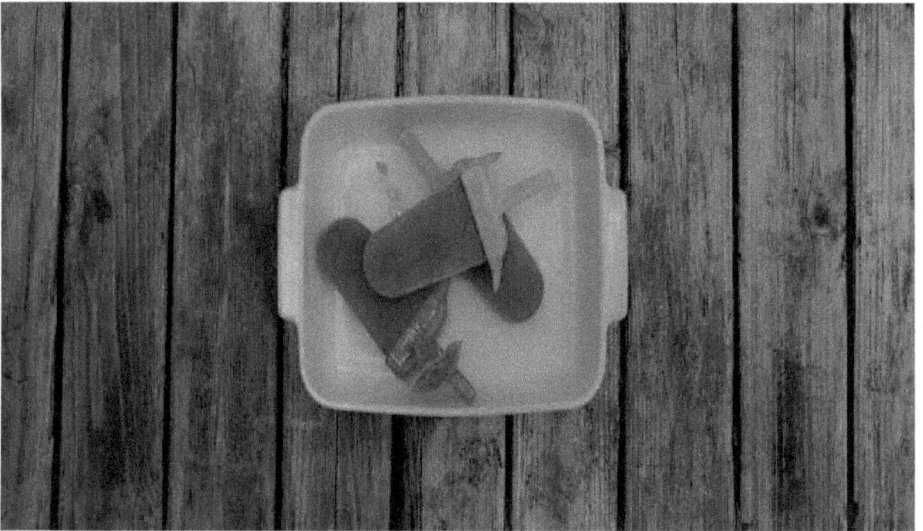

Dark Chocolate Mousse

Preparation Time: 10 minutes
Cooking Time: 10 minutes
Servings: 4

Ingredients:

3.5oz unsweetened dark chocolate, grated
½ tsp. vanilla
1 tbsp. honey
2 cups Greek yogurt
¾ cup unsweetened almond milk

Directions:

1.Add chocolate and almond milk in a saucepan and heat over medium heat until just chocolate melted. Do not boil.

2.Once the chocolate and almond milk combined then add vanilla and honey and stir well.

3.Add yogurt in a large mixing bowl.

4.Pour chocolate mixture on top of yogurt and mix until well combined.

5.Pour chocolate yogurt mixture into the serving bowls and place in refrigerator for 2 hours.

6.Top with fresh raspberries and serve.

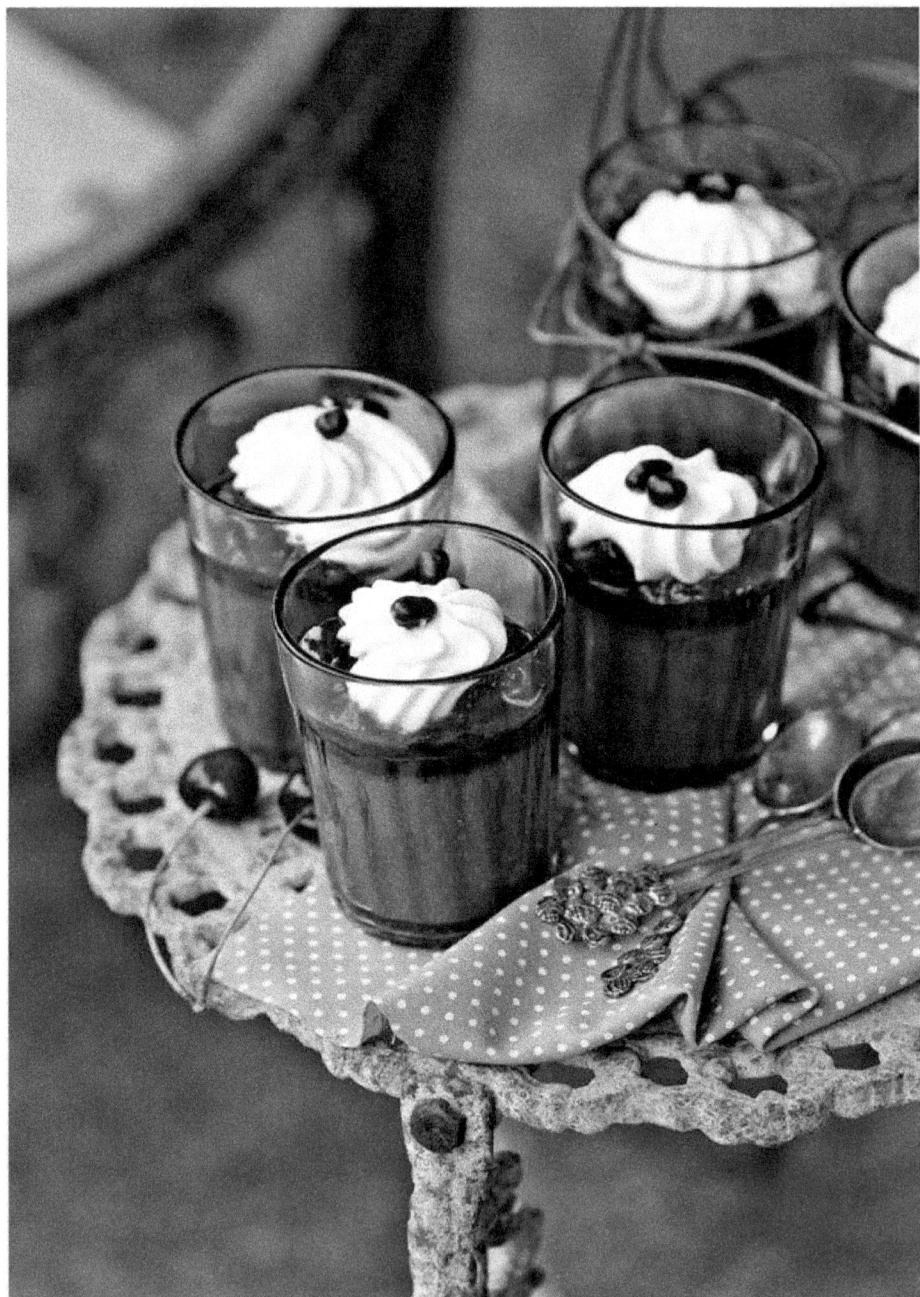

Warm & Soft Baked Pears

Preparation Time: 10 minutes

Cooking Time: 25 minutes

Servings: 4

Ingredients:
4 pears, cut in half and core
½ tsp. vanilla
¼ tsp. cinnamon
½ cup maple syrup

Directions:

1. Preheat the oven to 375°F.

2. Spray a baking tray with cooking spray.

3. Arrange pears, cut side up on a prepared baking tray and sprinkle with cinnamon.

4. In a small bowl, whisk vanilla and maple syrup and drizzle over pears.

5. Bake pears in preheated oven for 25 minutes.

6. Serve and enjoy.

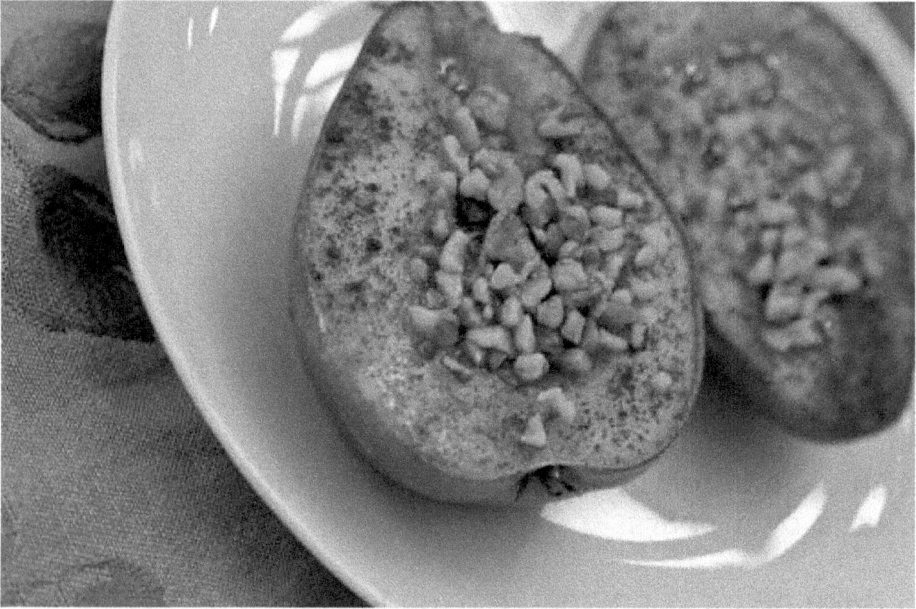

www.ingramcontent.com/pod-product-compliance
Lightning Source LLC
Chambersburg PA
CBHW050749030426
42336CB00012B/1723